In: Hunger and Poverty: Causes, Impacts and Eradication

HUNGER IN AMERICA: ISSUES AND ASSISTANCE

HUNGER AND POVERTY: CAUSES, IMPACTS AND ERADICATION

Hunger in America: Issues and Assistance
Gaston T. LaBue
2009 ISBN 978-1-60692-803-5

In: Hunger and Poverty: Causes, Impacts and Eradication

Hunger in America: Issues and Assistance

Gaston T. LaBue
Editor

Nova Science Publishers, Inc.
New York

For permission to use material from this book please contact us:
Telephone 631-231-7269; Fax 631-231-8175
Web Site: http://www.novapublishers.com

LIBRARY OF CONGRESS CATALOGING-IN-PUBLICATION DATA

ISBN: 978-1-60692-803-5

Published by Nova Science Publishers, Inc. ✢ New York

CONTENTS

PREFACE

The nutrition title of the omnibus 2008 "farm bill" is the focus of legislation affecting domestic food assistance programs in the 110th Congress. The program areas that are addressed include the regular Food Stamp program, programs operating in lieu of food stamps (e.g., Puerto Rico, Indian reservations), The Emergency Food Assistance Program (TEFAP), the Commodity Supplemental Food Program, Community Food Projects, the Seniors Farmers' Market Nutrition Program, initiatives to provide fresh fruit and vegetable in schools, and newly proposed nutrition and health promotion or support projects. Other nutrition programs (child nutrition and WIC programs) have not been a major part of the active legislative debate, although a number of bills noted in this new book address them, and some legislative changes affecting them are part of appropriations law and the farm bill.

The 2008 farm bill has been enacted as P.L. 110-246. The nutrition title of this law has a projected new cost of about $3 billion over the next 5 years (FY2008- FY2012) and well over $9 billion over the next 10 years (FY2008-FY2017). The major share of this spending is due to changes in food stamp rules — increasing benefits and loosening eligibility standards — and expansion of support for TEFAP and fresh fruit and vegetable initiatives.

The most significant substantive nutrition program issues that were raised in the farm bill debate were those surrounding the Food Stamp program and support for fruit and vegetable programs, particularly how much to add in new spending. Despite cost differences, the House and Senate bills were very similar in the policy changes they proposed. Their nutrition titles (Title IV) renamed the Food Stamp program, increased program benefits, and loosened some eligibility rules. They increased spending for TEFAP, added support for the fresh fruit and vegetable program, and allowed exercise of geographic preference when procuring food for child nutrition programs. However, they differed in some policy aspects. The House proposed substantial limits on states' ability to "privatize" their administration of food stamps (not adopted in the final measure). And the Senate's bill included a number of initiatives not covered in the House (only some of which were incorporated in the final law) relating to food stamp eligibility for able-bodied adults without dependents, eased access to the Food Stamp program, support for farmers' markets, projects to promote health and nutrition through the Food Stamp program, and dietary supplements.

A lingering issue involves the response of food assistance programs to recent, relatively rapid, food price inflation, although no legislation has been introduced in this regard.

In: Hunger in America: Issues and Assistance
Editor: Gaston T. LaBue, pp. 1-6

ISBN: 978-1-60692-803-5

Chapter 1

THE EFFECTS OF HUNGER AND FOOD INSECURITY IN AMERICA. SUBMITTED TO: SUBCOMMITTEE ON DEPARTMENT OPERATIONS, OVERSIGHT, NUTRITION, AND FORESTRY U.S. HOUSE COMMITTEE ON AGRICULTURE

James D. Weill*

Chairman Baca and Members of the Subcommittee, I am Jim Weill, President of the Food Research and Action Center, and we deeply appreciate the opportunity to testify at this important hearing today.

We greatly appreciate as well the work you did to produce an excellent nutrition title in the Farm Bill over the past 18 months; and we applaud your leadership in taking up so quickly the important concern of what remains to be done to address hunger in America and its harmful effects.

Before talking about the effects of hunger on the people of this country, I would like to discuss very briefly the extent of hunger and food insecurity. It is, after all, only because the problems of hunger and food insecurity are so unnecessarily widespread in our country that the effects are so significant for children and for adults, for our nation's health and educational systems and outcomes, for our nation's productivity, and for the economy as a whole and our fiscal well-being.

The latest official poverty data and hunger data from the Census Bureau and the U.S. Department of Agriculture are for 2006, and they tell us that, even as the economy grew in the early part of this decade, lower-income Americans were receiving a shrinking share of the economic pie. Because of inadequate wages and economic supports, the number of people living in poverty rose from 31.6 million in 2000 to 36.5 million in 2006. The number of people living in households facing food insecurity – the government phrase for families without

* James D. Weill: 1875 Connecticut Avenue, NW; Suite 540; Washington, DC 20009; (202) 986-2200; www.frac.org

the resources to feed themselves enough, or unable for economic reasons to purchase a healthy diet, or otherwise struggling with hunger – rose from 31 million in 1999 to 35.5 million in 2006. More than 12 million of the people living in food insecure households were children.

The problem not only has been getting broader, it has been getting deeper: almost all of the growth in food insecurity from 1999 to 2006 was in the most severe sub-category, what USDA now calls "very low food insecurity" (and which was known, until two years ago, as "food insecure with hunger"). The number of people in households in this most severe sub-category rose from 7.8 million in 1999 to 11.1 million in 2006.

Almost certainly the numbers are considerably worse today. For much of the last year the economic data have been dominated by rising food and energy prices, stagnant or declining wages, and growing unemployment, as well as severe housing problems. The food insecurity numbers described earlier were for 2006. There is little doubt that the 2007 data, which will be released in November, will be worse, and that the data for 2008, which we will not see released for another 16 months, will be worse still.

There are interventions needed now to mitigate the impacts of wider and deeper food insecurity caused by the current inflation and economic downturn. The suffering of families has deepened considerably. For example, the Food Research and Action Center estimates that the monthly cost of the Thrifty Food Plan (the food stamp market basket) has grown by $40 for a family of four since food stamp benefits were last adjusted for inflation – a huge impact on low-income families that already had inadequate resources to purchase a healthy diet.

Most important, in the short run, is the need for a temporary boost in food stamp benefits. This not only will help low-income families grapple with weak economic conditions, including rapidly rising food prices, but also will provide real economic stimulus to the nation's economy. Dollar for dollar there is no better stimulus expenditure than food stamp benefits because they get into the economy so fast: USDA and the states can get them quickly onto beneficiaries' Electronic Benefit Transfer cards, and hard-pressed beneficiaries will spend the boost quickly. This has been noted in the last six months by economists and budget experts ranging from Martin Feldstein to Robert Rubin, and from Ben Bernanke to Peter Orszag.[1] It is essential that a significant increase in food stamp help be part of any forthcoming economic stimulus or economic recovery package.

But we also must recognize that this nation had intolerably high levels of food insecurity before the economic downturn and escalating food price inflation, and will have them after economic recovery unless we focus on long-term solutions as well.

Long-term solutions are essential because the damage from hunger and food insecurity to individuals and families, to schools and the health care system, and to our economy as a whole is so great. I am just going to summarize how the harms play out, and then focus briefly on a couple of particular points.

- *Maternal undernutrition can impair body, organ and cellular growth in the fetus;* increases the risk of certain birth defects; and contributes to low infant birthweight, which is strongly correlated with perinatal and infant mortality.
- *Food insecurity among very young children can cause stunted growth, iron* deficiency anemia and delayed cognitive development. Cognitive delays then can last well

beyond the period of nutritional deficiency – the resulting impaired IQ, motor skills and coordination can last into the elementary school years and beyond.

- Food insecurity harms children's physical growth and immune systems, and causes weakened resistance to infection. Food insecure children are far more likely to be reported in poor health, to catch colds, and to have stomach aches, headaches, ear infections and asthma.
- *Food insecurity in both early childhood and the school years means that children lag their peers and learn less, and these learning deficits cumulate. School-age* children who are food insecure are more likely to be absent from school, be hyperactive; behave poorly; be held back; do worse on tests; and be placed in special education.

All of these consequences of hunger and food insecurity result in increased health, mental health, hospitalization, educational, juvenile justice and other costs. As just one example, among children under age 3, according to one study, those who are food insecure are 90 percent more likely to be in poor health and 30 percent more likely to require hospitalization.

For adults as well, there is a broad range of adverse outcomes of food insecurity. Some of them carry over from childhood. But food insecurity during the adult years independently means lower productivity and, as is true with children, means more doctor visits, higher rates of hospitalization and longer hospital stays, and poorer health.

Adult hunger and food insecurity also harm the children in the household. Two examples show how not only does hunger harm adults and children, but also how children will suffer even when adults bear the brunt and the children have enough to eat. One example involves depression, anxiety and stress; the other, overweight and obesity.

Often both of the parents or the single custodial parent in a household do everything they can to protect the children from the direct consequences of food insecurity or hunger: the children eat first, and get "enough" to eat (it may be filling but not be an adequate, healthy diet because of the resource constraints). But the parents are often hungry or skipping meals to protect the children. The resulting stress and depression with which food insecurity is associated harm not only the parents but the children's health and mental proficiency. Food insecurity adversely affects parent-child relationships.

One survey of several thousand mothers of 3-year old children in 18 large cities found that mental health problems in mothers and behavioral problems in their preschool-aged children were twice as likely in food insecure households as in food secure households. In discussing their findings, the researchers assert: "Social policy can address food insecurity more directly than it can address many other early-life stresses, and doing so can enhance the well-being of mothers and children."

As to obesity, research has shown that obesity too can be a consequence of food insecurity. Obesity among both adults and children means more cardiovascular disease, diabetes, and hypertension. Among adult food insecure women who have children, the reasons for obesity may include the ways in which low-income mothers must cope with limited resources for food—sacrificing at times their own nutrition in order to protect their children from hunger and lower nutritional quality. Food insecurity and poverty may also act as physiological stressors leading to hormonal changes that predispose adult women to obesity.

But there are connections between food insecurity and obesity for children as well. Children in food insecure households are more likely to be at risk of overweight or to be obese. When children are both born at low birthweight and live in a family suffering from food insufficiency, they have a 27.8 times higher chance of being overweight or obese at age 4 1/2 .

Finally, we must not forget that food insecurity harms seniors. Food insecure elderly persons have been found to be 2.33 times more likely to report fair or poor health status. And food insecurity among elders increases disability, decreases resistance to infection, and extends hospital stays. Moreover, many medications need to be taken with food to assure their effectiveness. Too many seniors have to skip meals in order to purchase medication, only to see a "Take with food" label on the prescription bottle because without food the drug will be less effective. Medically this is self-defeating, and, ultimately, costly. And from the patients' perspective it is a cruel "Catch-22."

What all this comes down to is that hunger and food insecurity not only are unnecessary and immoral in our wealthy nation, but they are vastly counter-productive in every important realm. They are a hindrance to our accomplishment of a range of essential national goals:

- *At a time when the nation is looking for strategies to broaden health insurance coverage and improve quality of health care while controlling costs, eliminating* food insecurity is a necessary part of an effective and cost-effective national health strategy.
- *As the nation struggles to address its obesity epidemic, establishing food security* and assuring that families have resources adequate to purchase a healthy diet are essential components of a successful anti-obesity strategy.
- At a time when our scientific knowledge of the critical importance of early *childhood development has been growing by leaps and bounds – although our policy development is having trouble keeping pace – eliminating food insecurity* is a prerequisite to the strongest possible early childhood policy.
- *As the nation struggles with education policy and the reauthorization of the No Child Left Behind Act, eliminating food insecurity is a compelling and cost-* effective strategy to improve schools and student performance.
- And as we struggle to restore economic growth, boost productivity, improve our *competitiveness, and keep deficits under control, eliminating food insecurity is one important key to improving the nation's economic and fiscal futures.*

It is essential that we address hunger and food insecurity in this nation and thereby eliminate the harms they cause. The Food Stamp Program and other federal nutrition programs have brought the nation a long way; and the recent Farm Bill made some important improvements in the Food Stamp Program. Again, we thank you, Mr. Chairman, and the Subcommittee, for your leadership in accomplishing this. But the Food Stamp Program (or, as it will be known from October 1st, the Supplemental Nutrition Assistance Program, or SNAP) in particular must be strengthened further so we can truly move towards eradicating hunger and food insecurity in the midst of our great affluence.

This requires three broad strategies: making benefit allotments adequate; opening eligibility to more needy people; and connecting more eligible people with benefits, since only

65 percent of currently eligible people, and barely half of eligible low-income working families, participate in the program.

Food stamps alone can't end hunger in this country – we also need stronger cash programs for economic security (refundable tax credits, unemployment insurance and other investments) and stronger child nutrition programs (school meals, WIC, summer and afterschool food, child care food). But food stamps are the critical base of the anti- hunger strategy.

Let me first address the pre-eminent need – to make benefit allotments more adequate. Food stamps are extraordinarily effective for families, but allotments just aren't enough to sustain health and well-being. It is the norm rather than the exception for a food stamp recipient household's benefits to run out several days before the end of the month - - often in the third week of the month. The Thrifty Food Plan, which is the underlying structure for the benefit amounts, has never represented what a family needs to purchase a minimally adequate diet, other than on an emergency basis. This shortfall of benefits was bad enough before, but it has been exacerbated by program changes in the 1980s and 1990s that, through several negative actions, cut benefits. (One 1996 change, freezing the standard deduction from income, was fixed prospectively by this year's Farm Bill; but much of the damage that the 1996 law and earlier changes have caused to benefit levels remains unremedied. As just two examples: benefits used to be adjusted for inflation twice a year, but now it is only once a year, which is particularly damaging in times of high inflation; and maximum benefit allotments were cut across the board by three percent in 1996.)

As this nation seeks to reduce the effects of hunger and food insecurity, *adequate food stamp allotments* are essential. SNAP benefits should be based on a food plan that reflects what it actually costs to feed a family a healthy diet, and the income counting rules that determine what share of a full allotment a family gets should be based in current economic realities.

The nation will need as well to have the program reach more low-income people. This means removing some arbitrary barriers to access for very needy people that are still in federal law. But it also means better efforts, at all levels of government, to connect already *eligible* people to benefits.

Only 65 percent of eligible people actually receive food stamp benefits. In many states, cities, towns and rural areas the number is far worse, because there is too much red tape, or too little outreach, or state and local rules narrow and discourage participation. Last autumn the Food Research and Action Center released a report on Food Stamp Access in Urban America. That analysis found that in 2007, in the 24 cities we looked at, the estimated rates of participation ranged from a low of 35 percent in San Diego, California to 98 percent in Detroit (Wayne County), Michigan. Three of the cities and counties with the lowest rates were in California – San Diego, Los Angeles, and Oakland (Alameda County).

When states or cities, or any areas, forego food stamp benefits, it harms low-income people. But it also harms local economies. USDA has found that every dollar of food stamp benefits, paid for by the federal government, that enters a community produces nearly twice that much in economic activity. In other words, there is nearly a 2:1 multiplier effect. The food stamp benefits not only, therefore, reduce hunger and poverty, but they create jobs and other economic benefits that further combat hunger and poverty and boost the community economy.

But states and cities are foregoing many billions of these dollars. Our 24-city study, for example, found that the cities were leaving $2.27 billion in federally-funded food stamp benefits unclaimed.

The cost of hunger and food insecurity to individuals, families, communities and the nation is far too high to continue to tolerate these and other losses. It is too high a cost in terms of health, education, productivity, mental health, economic growth, and community development. It is within this nation's capacity to end hunger and food insecurity. We look forward to working together with the members of the Subcommittee to make a stronger, more adequate and more accessible SNAP program a far more reliable bulwark against hunger in America.

REFERENCES

[1] These and other statements can be found at www.realstimulus.org

In: Hunger in America: Issues and Assistance
Editor: Gaston T. LaBue, pp. 7-65
ISBN: 978-1-60692-803-5

Chapter 2

DOMESTIC FOOD ASSISTANCE: THE FARM BILL AND OTHER LEGISLATION IN THE 110TH CONGRESS*

Joe Richardson

ABSTRACT

The nutrition title of the omnibus 2008 "farm bill" is the focus of legislation affecting domestic food assistance programs in the 110th Congress. The program areas that are addressed include the regular Food Stamp program, programs operating in lieu of food stamps (e.g., Puerto Rico, Indian reservations), The Emergency Food Assistance Program (TEFAP), the Commodity Supplemental Food Program, Community Food Projects, the Seniors Farmers' Market Nutrition Program, initiatives to provide fresh fruit and vegetable in schools, and newly proposed nutrition and health promotion or support projects. Other nutrition programs (child nutrition and WIC programs) have not been a major part of the active legislative debate, although a number of bills noted in this report address them, and some legislative changes affecting them are part of appropriations law and the farm bill.

The 2008 farm bill has been enacted as P.L. 110-246. The nutrition title of this law has a projected new cost of about $3 billion over the next 5 years (FY2008- FY20 12) and well over $9 billion over the next 10 years (FY2008-FY2017). The major share of this spending is due to changes in food stamp rules — increasing benefits and loosening eligibility standards — and expansion of support for TEFAP and fresh fruit and vegetable initiatives.

The most significant substantive nutrition program issues that were raised in the farm bill debate were those surrounding the Food Stamp program and support for fruit and vegetable programs, particularly how much to add in new spending. Despite cost differences, the House and Senate bills were very similar in the policy changes they proposed. Their nutrition titles (Title IV) renamed the Food Stamp program, increased program benefits, and loosened some eligibility rules. They increased spending for TEFAP, added support for the fresh fruit and vegetable program, and allowed exercise of geographic preference when procuring food for child nutrition programs.

* Excerpted from CRS Report RL33829, dated August 22, 2008.

However, they differed in some policy aspects. The House proposed substantial limits on states' ability to "privatize" their administration of food stamps (not adopted in the final measure). And the Senate's bill included a number of initiatives not covered in the House (only some of which were incorporated in the final law) relating to food stamp eligibility for able-bodied adults without dependents, eased access to the Food Stamp program, support for farmers' markets, projects to promote health and nutrition through the Food Stamp program, and dietary supplements.

A lingering issue involves the response of food assistance programs to recent, relatively rapid, food price inflation, although no legislation has been introduced in this regard.

This report will be updated as warranted by legislative action.

INTRODUCTION

In the 110th Congress, legislative action on virtually all domestic food assistance issues outside the annual Agriculture appropriations measures has been focused on the omnibus "farm bill" — periodic legislation (the last farm bill was enacted in 2002) that covers most programs and activities carried out by the U.S. Department of Agriculture (USDA or "Agriculture Department" in this report). Farm bills serve as a vehicle for reauthorizing a wide range of expiring authorities, making changes in (or ending) existing programs, and launching new initiatives.[1]

On the other hand, some food assistance efforts are reauthorized and reviewed on a different schedule and are up for review in 2009; these include child nutrition programs (like the School Lunch program), the Special Supplemental Nutrition Program for Women, Infants, and Children (the WIC program), and the WIC Farmers' Market Nutrition program.[2] With exceptions, annual appropriations laws typically are not the arena for significant policy decisions relating to nutrition assistance programs.[3] And some important nutrition program changes now under way at the USDA are unlikely to become the subject of legislation per se, such as revision of the content of food packages distributed through the WIC program, revamping the nutrition guidelines for school meals, modification of food packages offered under the Food Distribution Program on Indian Reservations (the FDPIR).

This report covers issues and legislative changes addressed in the farm bill, legislative changes included in the FY2008 Agriculture appropriations measure (included in the FY2008 Consolidated Appropriations Act; P.L. 110-161), and proposed legislation that involves programs and activities that are normally not part of the farm bill (e.g., child nutrition program proposals).

THE 2008 FARM BILL

Background

In FY2006, the $35 billion spent for federal programs and activities covered by the nutrition title of the 2002 farm bill (and addressed in the most recent farm bill) accounted for over half of the spending projected for all farm-bill-covered programs and activities and 36% of USDA outlays.[4] The lion's share of this support was for the Food Stamp program, which (along with child nutrition and WIC programs) is widely viewed as the federal government's primary response to the food needs of low-income Americans. Nutrition assistance programs also play a role in federal support for the agricultural sector through direct commodity purchases and increased demand for food.

The USDA oversees almost 20 domestic nutrition assistance programs and related activities, spending some $54 billion in FY2006, 55% of USDA outlays.[5] Virtually all are administered by states, schools, or local grantees under federally prescribed rules. Federal oversight of these programs (e.g., regulations governing program operations) is the responsibility of the USDA's Food and Nutrition Service (FNS). In addition, the USDA's Agricultural Marketing Service (AMS), the Farm Service Agency (FSA), and the Commodity Credit Corporation (CCC) play roles in the procurement and distribution of food commodities for some programs.

The farm bill covers 8 of these program areas accounting for about 65% of federal spending on domestic nutrition aid. Farm bills traditionally reauthorize expiring authorities and appropriations for these domestic nutrition assistance initiatives and are the principal vehicle for revising rules that govern how they operate and how much they will cost. They regularly include the following 5 area

- the regular Food Stamp program in the 50 states, the District of Columbia, Guam, and the Virgin Islands;
- programs operating in lieu of the regular Food Stamp program — nutrition assistance block grants for Puerto Rico, American Samoa, and the Northern Mariana Islands, along with the Food Distribution Program on Indian Reservations (the FDPIR);
- The Emergency Food Assistance Program (TEFAP);
- the Commodity Supplemental Food Program (the CSFP); and
- Community Food Projects.

Moreover, the 2002 farm bill added 3 items to this list. It provided statutory authority and mandatory funding for a new *Seniors Farmers' Market Nutrition Program* (the SFMNP) and established a pilot program to distribute *free fruits and vegetables in schools* (later expanded and made permanent). It also included a provision affecting commodities distributed to schools — earmarking some federal spending on these commodities for fresh produce acquired and distributed through Defense Department procurement facilities (the *"DOD Fresh" program*).

All farm bill domestic nutrition assistance programs, except for the CSFP, the FDPIR, and the administrative and distribution-cost component of TEFAP, generally are treated as *mandatory entitlements* for budget purposes. For the regular Food Stamp program, this means that, in order to affect costs, eligibility, benefit, or other program rules must be changed. Specific annual mandatory funding levels are set by law for the Puerto Rico and American Samoa grants (these are indexed), the food component of TEFAP, Community Food Projects, the SFMNP, and fresh fruit and vegetable projects. The amount of the Northern Marianas' grant is negotiated between the USDA and the Commonwealth. And decisions made with each year's appropriation govern the CSFP, the administrative and distribution cost component of TEFAP, and the amount set aside for the FDPIR.

The 2002 farm bill made extensive changes to Food Stamp program rules and relatively minor revisions to those for the other programs.[6] Using its March 2002 "baseline," the

Congressional Budget Office (CBO) estimated that the total additional cost of the provisions in the nutrition assistance title of the 2002 farm bill would be about $3 billion over the six-year life of the bill, representing 5%-6% of total new spending prompted by the bill. However, while there is no direct measure of the real cost of the 2002 bill's nutrition title (as opposed to costs incurred because of other variables like unforeseen participation changes related to economic conditions or increased participation rates), *total* actual costs through FY2005 for the programs covered by the nutrition title — including both "baseline" spending and new spending caused by the farm bill — were 12% higher than projected in 2002. If current CBO estimates for FY2006 and FY2007 are added in and compared to the 2002 estimates for those years, the gap widens to 20%.

Food Stamps[7]

The largest of the nutrition assistance programs is the Food Stamp program. At $33 billion in FY2006, it represents some 95% of the federal spending for farm bill nutrition assistance programs, is the foundation of federal initiatives to give low- income households the chance to obtain at least a minimally adequate diet, and is a major factor in overall federal policy for the poor.

The purpose (and structure) of the program has evolved over time. It is meant to play a role in three areas of federal public policy. Food stamps originated as a way of providing an outlet for surplus agricultural production, with the notable side benefit of supporting poor families. However, its goals and role in the country's support system for the low-income population have shifted and expanded greatly. To the extent it expands food purchasing power, it continues to support demand for agricultural products.[8] But it now also is seen as the government's primary response to important concerns about the overall "food security" status of the low-income population, although only an estimated 65% of eligible individuals choose to participate by the most recent count (2005). A 2006 Economic Research Service (ERS) study reports that, in 2005, 11% of U.S. households were "food insecure," and that the prevalence of "very low food security" was 3.9%.[9] Finally, the Food Stamp program has become an integral part of the overall "safety net" for the needy. It ranks as the fourth largest needs-tested program, behind Medicaid, the Earned Income Tax Credit, and the Supplemental Security Income program. It is perhaps the largest on-going program providing immediate aid to those affected by natural and other disasters. According to the USDA's Economic Research Service, when its benefits are added to other income, food stamps are estimated to move almost 10% of recipients out of poverty, and, for a typical low-income recipient family with children, food stamps can provide some 25% of their purchasing power.

Program Operation

The regular Food Stamp program provides inflation- indexed monthly benefits to low-income households that supplement their own spending on food; benefits vary by income, household expenses (like shelter costs), and household size — but generally not by state or region.[10] They are delivered through electronic benefit transfer (EBT) cards that are used like debit cards. Eligibility for food stamps is primarily based on a household's financial status. Monthly gross income typically must be below 130% of the inflation-indexed federal poverty income guideline for the household's size (e.g., $1,107 for a 1-person household and $1,861 for 3 persons in FY2008), and liquid assets must be under $2,000 ($3,000 for those households with elderly and disabled members). However, some households can be "categorically eligible" if they participate in or receive services under another income-tested program like Temporary Assistance for Needy Families (TANF) or the Supplemental Security Income (S SI) program. And certain categories are barred irrespective of their financial need, such as many noncitizens, able-bodied adults without dependents (ABAWDs) not meeting a work test.

Program costs are shared with the states, which administer the program under generally uniform federal rules. The federal government pays the full cost of benefits and about half the cost of administration, operating work or training programs for recipients, and state-directed nutrition education and outreach activities. States, and in some cases localities, pay the remainder (some $2.7 billion in FY2006).

The level of food stamp spending varies with participation, which is closely linked to economic conditions and eligibility rules, and benefit levels. Benefits are indexed to food-cost inflation and adjusted for recipients' income, household size, and certain nonfood expenses (like high shelter costs, child care spending); in addition, a basic (unindexed) minimum amount (the "standard deduction," typically $134 a month for each household) is disregarded when calculating a household's ability to contribute to its food needs. The basic theory underpinning food stamp benefits is that they should provide the difference between what a recipient household can afford for food out of its own monthly cash income (assumed to be about 30% of counted income) and the estimated minimal cost of an adequate diet (the monthly cost of the USDA's "Thrifty Food Plan" for its size). Since the 2002 farm bill, participation has increased substantially, from some 19 million persons per month in FY2002 to 27.2 million (October 2007), and the average monthly benefit level has jumped from $80 a person in FY2002 to $101 in October 2007.[11] Federal costs have grown from $20.6 billion in FY2002 to an estimated $33 billion for FY2007.

Finally, the Food Stamp program has a "quality control" system that measures the degree to which eligibility and benefit decisions are erroneously made. The most recent national quality control statistics (for 2005) show historically low error rates: 4.5% of benefits over-issued and 1.3% under-issued.[12] States with persistently high error rates can be assessed financial sanctions; those achieving high performance criteria can receive bonus payments.

Issues and Proposals

The 2002 farm bill reauthorized expiring Food Stamp program authorities and appropriations through FY2007. It greatly expanded eligibility for noncitizens (most notably allowing eligibility for noncitizen children and those who meet a five-year legal residence requirement), raised benefits modestly for larger households (by counting less of their income), and allowed states to provide "transitional" food stamps for families leaving the Temporary Assistance for Needy Families (TANF) program. In addition, the 2002 bill set up a number of state options to ease access to the program and administrative burdens on applicants and recipients and program operators (e.g., allowing states to reduce recipient reporting requirements, simplify benefit calculations, conform some food stamp rules to those used in the TANF and Medicaid programs) and revamped the quality control system to reduce the number of states subject to financial sanctions and grant bonus payments to states demonstrating exemplary administrative performance.[13] Virtually no program cuts were made.

Even small changes to eligibility or benefit rules in a program as large as food stamps can bring on relatively large budget costs or savings. And, as with the 2002 farm bill, the ability to revise the Food Stamp program depends heavily on budget constraints at the time the farm bill is considered. Major issues that emerged in the House and Senate consideration of the farm bill, and the Administration's farm bill package, related to eligibility for food stamps (including the treatment of household assets), the use of food stamp benefits, benefit levels, state administration, and program access. Details of congressional action on these issues are covered at the end of this report (and touched on in the following discussion); the food stamp proposals in the Administration's package are addressed in each of the issue areas covered in the following outline.

Eligibility

Both loosening and tightening current rules governing the eligibility of *noncitizens* have been raised as potential changes to food stamp rules. Although no major legislation to further restrict noncitizens' eligibility was introduced, in the 109th Congress, the House of the bill implementing spending reductions to comply with the FY2006 budget reconciliation measure would have further limited eligibility for noncitizens. On the other hand, several bills called for ending existing limits on legally resident noncitizens. The farm bill did not address the issue of noncitizens' eligibility for food stamps.

States may make households participating in their TANF programs *categorically eligible* (automatically eligible) for food stamps, and most states make use of this option. The Administration contends that states have taken advantage of this rule and made those with financial resources above normal food stamp standards eligible, simply by providing some minimal TANF-linked services. And, to protect program integrity, it proposed to limit categorical eligibility to those TANF recipients getting *cash* aid, which presumably is subject to financial tests similar to or more stringent than food stamps. On the other hand, opponents of this view noted that many of the estimated 300,000 persons affected are receiving services (e.g., child care, transportation assistance for work) that help them keep working, that they still must have their benefit calculated under normal food stamp rules and can only qualify for a benefit if they have high living expenses (e.g., shelter costs), that limiting categorical eligibility would impose added administrative burdens on states and applicants, and that, as a side-effect, a number of children would lose eligibility for free school meals.[14] No legislation concerning categorical eligibility was introduced (and the farm bill did not address this issue), but it is important to remember that limiting categorical eligibility is one of very few proposals that put forward that would produce significant cost savings.

Opponents of the current restrictions on participation by *able-bodied adults without children (ABA WDs)*, which bar eligibility after three months unless the individual meets a work-related test, contend that they should either be abolished as too punitive (and administratively complex) or greatly eased. These restrictions were put in place as part of the 1996 welfare reform law, and, in many cases, they can be (and are) waived by states; although the Senate farm bill would have eased them, the enacted law did not.

Finally, the Administration proposed (1) new rules that would disqualify food stamp recipients who exchange food purchased with their benefits for cash or misuse benefits to obtain container deposits and bar from food stamps those who have been disqualified from the Food Distribution Program on Indian Reservations (the FDPIR) and (2) making permanent a rule disregarding combat pay when considering the eligibility of (and benefit amounts for) military households. The enacted farm bill contains similar provisions.

Assets

Current policy excludes most, but not all, retirement savings from consideration as assets when testing for food stamp eligibility. While the 2002 farm bill allowed states to expand the list of excluded retirement savings (e.g., to include Individual Retirement Accounts) under certain conditions, very few states have. In a similar vein, current food stamp policy disregards savings for education as assets only if a determination is made that they are "inaccessible." The Administration and others supported disregarding *all* tax-recognized retirement savings or plans and education savings to avoid penalizing those who save for retirement or education but are temporarily in need. The Food Stamp program's dollar asset limits have not been significantly changed in over 25 years. Program advocates argued that they should be raised (or possibly abolished) to encourage saving and simplify administration. In addition to the Administration's farm bill package, a number of bills dealing with loosening asset rules have been introduced. The enacted farm bill loosens asset rules along the line discussed above.

Use of Benefits

Food stamp benefits can be used for virtually any food purchase; they cannot be used for alcohol, tobacco, hot prepared food, or dietary supplements. Food choice has been a recurring theme in food stamp policy debates. Critics argue that nutrition-related limits should be placed on the types of food that can be bought with food stamps. On the other hand, others contend that incentives to purchase healthy foods should be built into the Food Stamp program and that support for nutrition education should be increased and expanded to cover a broader range of initiatives. Separately, some have proposed to allow food stamps to be used for dietary supplements, as in the Senate version of the 2002 farm bill. The Senate version of the 2007 farm bill included provisions that opened up the possibility that food stamp benefits could be used to purchase dietary supplements and included provisions for projects to encourage the use of food stamp benefits for healthful foods. The enacted farm bill does not include changes with regard to dietary supplements but does authorize efforts to support the purchase of healthful foods.

Benefit Levels

A major contention of critics of the current structure of the Food Stamp program has been that the value of food stamp benefits has been significantly "eroded" since the 1996 welfare reform law; that is, benefits are significantly smaller than they would have been without the changes made in 1996.[15] Although basic (maximum) food stamp benefits are indexed annually, they point out that rising non-food living costs are heavily affecting recipients' budgets (limiting their ability to supplement their food stamp benefits as the program expects) and that one of the program's major methods for taking these costs into account when calculating benefits (a uniform income disregard called the "standard deduction") has been effectively frozen (at $134 a month) since 1996. They also note that the 1996 law imposed an across-the-board 3% benefit cut. Program advocates, and a number of bills, aim to address this by increasing and indexing the standard deduction, raising maximum benefits by 3%, or both. Opponents of this type of action are concerned about the substantial costs involved and argue that the Food Stamp program should not be expected to be a general purpose income support program responding to all of the needs of the low-income population. The enacted farm bill addresses this issue with a boost to the standard deduction.

Separately, the Administration and several bills proposed to remove the current dollar limits on the degree to which dependent care expenses are considered when calculating benefits, thus increasing assistance for those with very high dependent care expenses related to work — as does the enacted farm bill.

Finally, as in earlier farm bill debates, there were proposals to increase and index the Food Stamp program's minimum benefit level ($10 a month for 1- and 2- person households). It has not been changed since originally set in the late 1970s and is seen as so low that it discourages participation, especially among the elderly. However, this relatively costly change would most help those in the program with the highest incomes. The enacted farm bill increases the minimum benefit.

State Administration

States (most notably Florida, Indiana, and Texas) have taken, or are taking, major steps to revamp the way they administer food stamps, Medicaid, and the TANF program.[16] Food stamp law requires that final eligibility and benefit decisions be made by government employees and that contracts for computer-related services with federal matching money be federally approved. However, these state initiatives can involve "privatizing" (contracting out or outsourcing) many "back-office" and other, more important administrative tasks and "modernizing and streamlining" administration through efforts like performing program intake by computer application and establishing "call centers" using private- sector employees, resulting in cost savings from fewer state staff and offices and, it is hoped, better client service. There are few federal standards for these types of initiatives (e.g., with respect to client service, pilot testing, what roles private company employees can play, how extensive displacement of government employees can be). Many of those watching the current initiatives have argued that standards should be set legislatively to give the federal government the ability to more effectively oversee the progress in this area or that limits should be placed on states' ability to delegate administrative responsibilities to non-state employees and entities. They point out that modernization and streamlining steps can potentially leave some vulnerable groups without real access to food stamp help, needlessly complicate the application and benefit process, blur lines of accountability, result in incorrect information for, or treatment of, applicants and recipients, and end many state jobs. However, a number of states are concerned that legislatively set privatization standards/limits will severely restrict innovation in administering food stamps and other public assistance programs and reduce or eliminate cost savings that might result. On the other hand, the Administration has been concerned about widespread benefit overpayments that can occur in a changeover to new administrative systems and would like to hold states (not recipients) responsible in cases of "widespread systemic errors."

The enacted farm bill includes a number of provisions for oversight of state changes in their systems for administering food stamps but does not have provisions substantially limiting "privatization" initiatives.

The Food Stamp program's quality control system for overseeing state administration also is under some scrutiny. The Administration proposed two important changes: (1) impose financial penalties on states with high rates of error in denying food stamp benefits and (2) end an option for states to "invest" amounts owed as financial penalties for high rates of error in overissuing or underissuing benefits in administrative improvements as an alternative to paying part of their fiscal sanction to the federal government. Others would increase bonus payments to states meeting high performance standards. The enacted farm bill includes no changes in the quality control system.

Program Access

The participation rate among food stamp eligibles has increased since 2002 (when a number of changes were put in place to encourage this). However, with the most recently reported rate at 65% (2005), program advocates have argued that further steps need to be taken. In their view, procedural rules governing how applicants and recipients are treated (e.g., reporting requirements), as well as those relating to eligibility for applicants participating in other public assistance programs, could be further loosened to *ease access to food stamp benefits*. For example, added federal administrative cost-sharing for access-oriented state administrative changes (e.g., longer office hours), grants for access-improving efforts, loosened reporting requirements, and changes in application procedures could be legislated. Moreover, advocates have been concerned about any access restrictions that might result from the initiatives to privatize, modernize, or streamline administration noted above.

In addition to issues surrounding applicants' access to food stamps, proposals from the Administration would change rules governing *food retailers' participation* in the Food Stamp program, such as revising rules governing fines imposed on retailers' violating food stamp rules.

The enacted farm bill incorporates a number of provisions dealing with program access issues and retailer participation questions.

Administration Food Stamp Initiatives[17]

In early 2007, the USDA advanced a number of recommendations for changes in the Food Stamp program as part of the 2007 farm bill; they were not introduced as a legislative package, and only a few have been adopted in the enacted 2008 farm bill.

- Eligibility. *The Administration proposed to restrict categorical* (automatic) eligibility for food stamps to households who receive cash Temporary Assistance for Needy Families (TANF) benefits; *those receiving only TANF-funded services would not be* automatically eligible (on the premise that cash benefit recipients are subject to stricter eligibility tests). This revision accounted for the bulk of savings attributed to its proposals for nutrition program changes. The Administration was especially concerned that states can, in effect, "game" the categorical eligibility option and make households with financial resources well above normal food stamp limits eligible for food stamps by simply providing minimal services financed with TANF funds. On the other hand, critics pointed out that the services being provided often are key to supporting households' work efforts (e.g., child care), that there would be added administrative costs to carry out full eligibility determinations for those who chose to apply through regular procedures, and that some households losing their categorical food stamp eligibility would, as a result, lose their food-stamp-participation-based automatic eligibility for free school meals for their children. The Administration also proposed to place into permanent food stamp law a rule disregarding combat-related military pay as income when determining eligibility (and benefits). This has been done through provisions of appropriations laws since the FY2005 Department of Agriculture appropriations act. However, some observers contended that better use of the Defense Department's special family assistance supplemental allowance program for military families might be a better way to deal with these families' needs. Finally, the Administration proposed new rules that would disqualify food stamp recipients who exchange food purchased with their benefits for cash or misuse benefits to obtain container deposits and those who have been barred from the Food Distribution Program on Indian Reservations (FDPIR). Only the combat-related pay, food purchase, and FDPIR proposals were picked up in the enacted farm bill.

- *Assets. The Administration proposed to disregard all retirement savings and plans and Internal Revenue Service (IRS)-approved* postsecondary education savings and plans as assets when judging food stamp eligibility. This proposal accounted for most of the cost of its nutrition program proposals. Its purposes are to reinforce federal policy encouraging savings for these ends and avoid penalizing those in temporary need who have put aside money for *retirement or education. However, some critics argued that asset* eligibility rules should be loosened even further than recommended by the Administration, for example, by raising or indexing the dollar limit on allowable assets or by standardizing the application of more liberal rules on how to count the value of households' vehicles. The enacted farm bill adopts the Administration's recommendations and raises dollar limits on allowable assets.
- *Benefit Levels. In order to support recipients' work and education* efforts, the Administration recommended removing limits on benefit increases that adjust for households' dependent care expenses — ending restrictions that do not take into account work — and education-related dependent care costs above $200 a month for each child under age 2 and $175 a month for all other dependents. *However, some critics argued that food stamps should not be viewed* as a "child care" program, while others maintained that there is a need to go further in recognizing the effect high non-food living expenses have in eroding the value of food stamps. The enacted farm bill incorporates the Administration's recommendation.
- *State Administration. The Administration advanced four revisions* to rules governing state administration of food stamps. It would assess states a quality control financial penalty if the state has a *"negative action" error rate above the national average for two* consecutive years; negative action error rates measure the extent to which states improperly deny, suspend, or terminate food stamp applicants and recipients.[18] Secondly, it proposed to eliminate an *option permitting states to invest in administrative improvements as* an alternative to paying part of any quality control fiscal sanction. In addition, in the case of "widespread systemic errors" (e.g., major computer system failures and flaws) in a state's administration of the program, the Administration proposed to (1) prohibit states from pursuing claims against recipients for over-issued benefits

and (2) require states to pay the federal government for the cost of over- issuances. Only the Administration recommendations with respect to systemic errors are addressed in the enacted farm bill.

- *Retailers Participation in the Program. With regard to retailers' participation in the Food Stamp program, the Administration argued* that it needs more flexibility to respond to the seriousness of a retailer's violation of program rules and would like, for example, *more authority to impose fines in lieu of disqualification for minor* violations and new authority to fine retailers in addition to *disqualification for major violations. It also advanced a proposal to* allow the Department of Agriculture to immediately suspend redemption of retailers' food stamp receipts (where expedited action is warranted) in "certain egregious trafficking cases." These retailer participation recommendations are covered in the enacted farm bill.
- *Other Proposals. The Administration's farm bill package would* have renamed the Food Stamp program the Food and Nutrition program, in recognition of the changes in how food stamp benefits *are delivered (i.e., through electronic benefit transfer systems) and* the program's role in improving nutrition.[19] It also would have *established a pilot project under which states would be allowed to* pay (with 50% federal matching) for state support for some work- related expenses incurred by working food stamp recipients. And it proposed to add specific language to the law referring to nutrition education as a major component of the Food Stamp program and as an approved activity for federal funding.[20] The enacted farm bill renames the Food Stamp program.

Programs in Lieu of Food Stamps

Four programs, three directly authorized in the Food Stamp Act, operate in lieu of food stamp assistance.

- *Puerto Rico receives an annual block grant indexed for food-price* inflation (about $1.5 billion at present, serving about 1 million persons per month) to operate a nutrition assistance program that works much like the regular Food Stamp program, including delivery *of benefits through EBT cards.[21] The major feature distinguishing* Puerto Rico's program from the regular Food Stamp program (other *than more restrictive financial eligibility tests and lower maximum benefit levels) is that just 75% of a household's benefit must be used for food purchases, as opposed to 100% in the regular Food Stamp* program. Puerto Rico was converted to its nutrition assistance block grant in 1982; as a quid pro quo, it was given total flexibility in how its program is designed.
- Since 1994, American Samoa has received an annual nutrition *assistance grant ($6.1 million in FY2006); it has designed a program* that serves low-income elderly and disabled persons (some 3,000 *persons in FY2005). This grant was established under the USDA's* discretionary authority to extend USDA programs to American Samoa and other territories, but is now funded under the same section of the Food Stamp Act as Puerto Rico's block grant and indexed like Puerto Rico's.

- Since 1982, the Commonwealth of the Northern Mariana Islands *has been provided an annual grant (negotiated with the USDA, with* an estimated $8.4 million available for FY2006) to operate a foodstamp-like program with 30% of benefits earmarked for locally produced products. This grant is authorized under P.L. 96-597 (a law governing relations with the Commonwealth) and, as such, has not in the past been part of a farm bill.
- *Indian tribal organizations may choose to operate the Food Distribution Program on Indian Reservations (FDPIR), instead of having the state offer regular food stamp benefits; the full cost of* benefits and most administrative expenses are covered by the federal government.[22] This option operates on over 250 Indian reservations in 22 states. The program offers nutritionally balanced monthly food packages of USDA-provided commodities to those meeting *eligibility rules close to those used for food stamps; households may* not get both food stamp and FDPIR benefits. It serves up to 100,000 persons per month at a cost of about $80 million (some 30% for administrative and distribution costs). The FDPIR distributes both commodities bought specifically for it ("entitlement" commodities) and "bonus" commodities acquired by the USDA for farm support reasons; the monthly value of the food packages averages $40-$45 a person.

Issues and Proposals

The 2002 farm bill extended through FY2007 the three programs now authorized under the Food Stamp Act: grants to Puerto Rico and American Samoa and the FDPIR.[23] It also slightly increased and indexed the nutrition assistance grants for Puerto Rico and American Samoa, and specifically authorized American Samoa's grant as part of the Food Stamp Act. Legislative issues related to these programs have been focused on Puerto Rico's nutrition assistance grant and the FDPIR.

Puerto Rico advocates argued that funding for assistance in Puerto Rico lags behind need. Bills in the House and Senate would increase Puerto Rico's nutrition assistance grant (and then index it for both food-cost inflation and population growth), require a study of the feasibility and effects of treating Puerto Rico as a state under the regular Food Stamp program, or both. Opponents are concerned over the costs associated with expansion of the grant and the prospect of having (potentially) over half the Commonwealth's population receiving aid. There were no Administration proposals (other than extending existing law) with regard to Puerto Rico. The enacted farm bill extends Puerto Rico's current indexed grant and directs a study of the effects and feasibility of treating Puerto Rico as a state for food stamp purposes.

Significant questions have been raised over the level of federal support for FDPIR costs for administration and distribution of commodities on Indian reservations and the degree to which funding for the FDPIR limits the types and quality of the foods provided. The Administration proposed a slight increase in the amount provided for FDPIR administrative and distribution costs in order to speed implementation of a new formula for allocating federal aid that is more directly tied to participation while easing the negative effects for tribal organizations that would lose money under the new allocation method. Others have called for a major increase in funding for FDPIR administrative and distribution expenses. In addition, some consideration is being given to boosting support for federal spending on the commodities provided through the FDPIR, and program advocates would like to see a thorough review of the adequacy and quality of FDPIR food packages and attention given to purchase of tribally produced foods. The enacted farm bill incorporates minor changes with regard to the FDPIR and calls for a review of the FDPIR food package.

The Emergency Food Assistance Program (TEFAP)[24]

TEFAP was begun in 198 1-1982 as a temporary expedient designed, at least initially, to dispose of huge stocks of government-held food commodities. It also occurred in the aftermath of noticeable reductions in the coverage of and benefits provided by food assistance programs like food stamps and school meal programs legislated in 198 1-1982, and in the midst of an economic recession and concern over "hunger" and homelessness among the needy. In 1983, the Emergency Food Assistance Act gave the program official status and authorized funding for administrative and distribution costs.

In the early years (through FY1988), the only significant federal expenditures involved were appropriations for administrative and distribution costs. The commodities were so-called "bonus" commodities, those acquired for farm-support reasons and held in excess of what was needed to fulfill other federal commitments (e.g., to school meal programs). The establishment of TEFAP helped reduce federal commodity stocks (and storage costs associated with them), provided an alternative source of food assistance for the needy, and was instrumental in supporting and expanding a network of emergency food aid providers that also drew food and other resources from many non-governmental sources.

In 1988, after the Administration indicated plans to phase out the program because of the lack of bonus commodity inventories, Congress began the practice of mandating funding for TEFAP commodities, thereby creating a minimum "entitlement" to a certain level of commodity assistance. This entitlement component was ensconced in permanent law by the 1996 welfare reform act (P.L. 104-193), which guaranteed the program $100 million a year. Additional bonus commodities continued to be made available — differing each year according to USDA acquisitions. This guarantee was increased to $140 million a year in the 2002 farm bill.

Under TEFAP, the federal government provides food commodities to states. This assistance supplements other sources of food aid for needy persons and often is provided in concert with food bank and homeless shelter projects, either as food packages or meals. Eligibility decisions for TEFAP assistance are made by states, and they choose local administering agencies. National emergency provider and food bank networks (like America's Second Harvest) also are heavily involved.

In addition to state allocations of the $140 million in entitlement commodities, each state receives a share of the $50 million a year appropriated as discretionary money to fund expenses associated with administration and distribution (storage, transportation) of the commodities, and states may divert some of the $140 million to administration and distribution costs.[25] Moreover, state entitlements to TEFAP commodities are supplemented with *bonus commodities* (about $150 million in FY2005) that the USDA has acquired in its agriculture support programs.

Issues and Proposals

The 2002 farm bill extended TEFAP authorities through FY2007 and increased the level of entitlement commodities from $100 million to $140 million a year. Since the 2002 farm bill, bonus commodity donations from USDA stocks to TEFAP have dropped dramatically — from over $240 million in FY2003 to about $150 million in FY2005, with estimates of less than $100 million for FY2006 and perhaps FY2007 and FY2008. Because USDA commodities provide an important underpinning to emergency food assistance providers' activities and they have come to rely on them, there are several proposals for the 2007 farm bill to substantially increase the level of entitlement commodity assistance above the current $140 million a year. The enacted farm bill greatly boosts the guaranteed level of TEFAP commodities.

Commodity Supplemental Food Program (CSFP)[26]

The CSFP was originally established in the late 1960s, under the authority of a series of appropriations laws, to provide aid to low-income women (pregnant and postpartum), infants, and children, who at that time had no other food assistance program to turn to for aid specific to their needs. Since then, the WIC program has largely taken over this role. However, the CSFP continues to operate and now serves mostly elderly low-income individuals who either need extra help beyond food stamp benefits or are reluctant to apply for food stamps. Projects supported by the CSFP typically provide a range of other services to their communities.

The CSFP provides supplemental foods to low-income elderly persons and low- income pregnant, postpartum, and breastfeeding women, infants, and children through over 140 projects in 32 states, the District of Columbia, and on two Indian reservations. For elderly participants, eligibility is limited to those with income below 130% of the federal poverty income guidelines (e.g., about $13,000 a year for 1 person); for households composed of women, infants, and children, the income ceiling is higher (185% of the poverty guidelines). The foods are purchased by the USDA and distributed to grantees, and food packages received and distributed by CSFP projects are designed with the specific nutritional needs of the elderly and women, infants, and children in mind. CSFP grantees also receive significant funding for administrative costs. The program is a discretionary program depending on annual appropriations decisions, and commodities and administrative funding generally are apportioned by the number of persons served in the prior year; if new money is appropriated or allocated "slots" are not used, new projects can be added. The commodities provided by the USDA are of two types: (1) "entitlement" commodities bought with annually appropriated funds and included in the food packages and (2) "bonus" commodities donated from USDA stocks and provided in addition to, or as part of, food packages.

In FY2005, the CSFP served some 500,000 persons a month, 90% of whom were elderly. Some $82 million in entitlement commodities and $38 million worth of bonus commodities were distributed; food packages were valued at between $18 and $21 per person per month. Administrative cost support was $29 million.

Issues and Proposals

The 2002 farm bill extended the authorization for the CSFP through FY2007 and increased the proportion of appropriations earmarked for administrative costs. In recent appropriations requests, the Administration has proposed terminating the CSFP, as duplicative of other programs (the WIC program and food stamps). However, neither House nor Senate Agriculture appropriations measures have adopted this position.[27] CSFP advocates have, for a number of years, called for a change in rules that would boost the income eligibility limit for the elderly from 130% of the federal poverty guidelines to 185% (the same as that applied to households with women, infants, and children). The enacted farm bill makes no significant changes to the CSFP.

Community Food Projects

In the 1996 farm bill, Congress established, as Section 25 of the Food Stamp Act (7 U.S.C. 2034), a program of assistance for community food projects, intended to promote innovative local self-help initiatives to meet nutrition and farm needs.

Community food projects are funded at a total of $5 million a year — a sum set aside from each year's Food Stamp Act appropriation. The program consists of competitive grants administered through the USDA's Cooperative State Research, Education, and Extension Service (CSREES), and requiring a 50% match.

Project grants provide one-time infusions of federal dollars for local projects designed to increase the food self-reliance of communities; promote comprehensive responses to local food, farm, and nutrition issues; develop innovative linkages among the public, for-profit, and nonprofit food sectors; encourage long-term planning and multi-agency approaches; or improve the availability of locally or regionally produced foods to low-income people. In addition, one special grant is mandated — to a non-governmental entity that coordinates and disseminates recommendations garnered from the various local projects.

Issues and Proposals

With little debate, the 2002 farm bill extended funding for community food projects through FY2007. Several measures before the 110th Congress would substantially increase funding for Community Food Projects, raise the federal share of projects' costs, expand the projects' scope, and raise the time limit on project grants. The enacted farm bill makes no major changes affecting community food projects.

Farmers' Market Nutrition Programs

Two farmer's market nutrition programs receive federal funding. The nutrition title of the 2002 farm bill provided statutory authority and mandatory funding (at $15 million a year through FY2007) for a new *Senior Farmers' Market Nutrition program (SFMNP)*, under which low-income seniors receive vouchers that they may redeem at farmers' markets and roadside stands for fresh produce. The SFMNP was set up to give low-income elderly the same help that women, infants, and children (WIC recipients) receive through WIC farmers' market vouchers. Separately, the *WIC farmers' market nutrition program* (authorized in child nutrition law and typically not part of the farm bill) provides vouchers for WIC recipients, with the level of support set by annual appropriations (typically about $20 million a year).

Issues and Proposals

Several legislative proposals would increase mandatory funding for the SFMNP and, for its WIC counterpart, increase funding and make it mandatory. The Administration proposed to (1) require that the value of SFMNP vouchers be disregarded in judging eligibility and benefits for federal and state means-tested aid and (2) prohibit states from participating in the SFMNP if state or local sales taxes are charged on the food purchased with SFMNP vouchers (as is already the case for the WIC farmers' market nutrition program). The enacted farm bill increases mandatory funding for the SFMNP and accepts the Administration's recommendations.

Finally, food stamp benefits can be used in approved farmers' markets, and several proposals for grants to help increase the number of participating farmers' markets (through technical assistance, infrastructure improvement, and training) have been advanced. These are primarily aimed at facilitating and expanding the use of food stamp electronic benefit transfer (EBT) cards at farmers' markets. The enacted farm bill includes funding for expansion of the use of food stamp electronic benefit transfer cards in farmers' markets.

Fruits and Vegetables

The nutrition title of the 2002 farm bill addressed, for the first time, the availability of fresh fruits and vegetables in schools — because of growing concerns over childhood obesity and the quality and types of foods offered through school meal programs. It established a pilot project under which a small number of elementary and secondary schools in a limited number of states and Indian reservations receive funding to offer free fresh fruit and vegetables to students.[28] The project was expanded, given mandatory annual funding, made permanent through the 2004 child nutrition reauthorization law (P.L. 108-265), and further expanded and given added money in P.L. 109-97. In FY2006-FY2007, about 400 schools in 14 states and 3 Indian reservations received support for this project, supported by funding totaling $15 million; this funding was used for activities covering both FY2006 and FY2007.

Separate from its nutrition title, the 2002 farm bill (in Section 10603) required that a minimum of $200 million a year in Section 32 funds be used to purchase "specialty crops" (like fruits and vegetables) and that $50 million a year of this amount be used for fresh fruit and vegetables acquired for school meal programs through the Defense Department procurement system, known as the DOD Fresh program.

Issues and Proposals[29]

Given concerns over obesity and the quality of government-provided commodities and school meals, there have been many initiatives relating to fruits and vegetables. The fresh fruit and vegetable program set up by the 2002 farm bill has proved popular; for example, both the House and Senate appropriations bills for FY2007 included an expansion in funding and the number of states covered. And the Administration's farm bill package, as well as several bills before Congress, would greatly expand the federal commitment to making more fruits and vegetables available through federally supported nutrition programs.

A number of bills would boost funding for the fresh fruit and vegetable program so that it could operate in all states (although not all schools). Some of the same bills would up the minimum required spending on fruits and vegetables (from Section 32 funds) to at least $400 million a year and increase the set-aside for the DOD Fresh program; most of these purchases would go to schools. The Administration proposed to provide new money, $50 million a year, for the purchase of fruits and vegetables specifically for the School Lunch program (above acquisitions under any other authority). It also supported increasing purchases of fruits and vegetables using Section 32 money by an escalating amount starting at $200 million a year and totaling $2.75 billion over 10 years.

Other initiatives include new funding for a fruit and vegetable promotion program, pilot projects offering financial incentives for food stamp recipients to purchase fruits and vegetables, grants to facilitate the procurement and transportation of highly perishable healthy foods for low-income persons, a proposal to require the Agriculture Department to establish its own program for acquiring fruits and vegetables for schools and allowing schools to divert a significant portion of their federal commodity "allowance" to purchase fruits and vegetables through the Department's program, and grants to community-based organizations and other local agencies to promote greater consumption of fresh fruits, vegetables, and other healthy foods in low-income communities.

The enacted 2008 farm bill incorporates a very substantial increase in funding for the program of free fresh fruits and vegetables in schools, so that it can operate nationally (although not in all schools). In addition, the FY2008 Agriculture Department Appropriations measure includes a small ($10 million) increase in funding for this program.

OTHER DOMESTIC FOOD ASSISTANCE ISSUES AND PROPOSALS

A number of proposals outside the scope of traditional farm bills also are before Congress, and many have been addressed in the 2008 farm bill (discussed later). In addition, one bill relating to nutrition support has been enacted (P.L. 110-19); this law makes clear that nutrition programs for the elderly operated under the authority of the *Older Americans Act* (home-delivered meals and congregate meal projects) may use their Older Americans Act funding to obtain food commodities for meals they serve through the Department of Agriculture.

The Administration has proposed a *pilot obesity initiative* that calls for competitive grants ($20 million a year over five years) to develop and test ways of addressing obesity in the low-income population, with evaluations of the results. According to the Department of Agriculture, ideas that might be tested include pointof-sale incentives for the purchase of fruits and vegetables by food stamp recipients, grants to connect food stamp shoppers with farmers' markets, and integrated communication and education programs to promote healthy diets and physical activity. Moreover, several bills call for similar projects. The

2008 farm bill (discussed later) includes provisions addressing projects similar to those proposed by the Administration.

Several bills, and the 2008 farm bill (discussed later) would encourage the purchase of locally produced foods by the Agriculture Department, the Defense Department, and nutrition program providers (e.g., schools). They would effectively override current rules that limit the extent to which the Departments, schools, and other providers can specify a *geographic (e.g. local) preference* when procuring food for donation or meals. Others would provide grants to support the work of food banks and similar nonprofit emergency feeding organizations related to obtaining, handling, storing, and distributing locally produced food.

A number of proposals include authorization for grants to community-based organizations for activities bolstering *food security* in their communities, as well as grants to national and regional groups to provide training and technical assistance. The 2008 farm bill (discussed later) contains similar authority.

Child nutrition program initiatives include the following:

- *providing mandatory funding for a currently authorized pilot project* for raising the income limit for free school meals to 185% of the federal poverty income guidelines;
- *authorizing a school breakfast program in which all meals are served* free, without regard to family income, in place of the current breakfast program;
- authorizing *start-up grants* for school breakfast programs;
- expanding the provision of federal child nutrition subsidies for dinners served in *after-school programs* to additional states.
- making simplified *summer food service program* rules nationally applicable.[30]
- changing "competitive foods" requirements by (1) mandating that *the current limited definition of "foods of minimal nutritional value"* be revised and expanded and (2) using this new definition to effectively bar selling these foods (sold in "competition" with school meal programs) on school campuses at any time during the school *day; and*
- establishing and funding a competitive grant program for schools to *create healthy school nutrition environments and assessing the effect of these environments on the health and well-being of their students.*
- *expanding the summer food service program by increasing the* number of areas in which free summer meals may be offered and providing start-up grants for new summer program sponsors.
- making nationally applicable rules (now used in a pilot project in Pennsylvania) that ease participation by *summer program sponsors in rural areas.*

Of the above-noted child nutrition proposals, only the initiatives making *simplified summer food service rules* nationally applicable and expanding subsidies for *dinners in after-school programs* to additional states have been acted on; the Agriculture Department's FY2008 appropriation (included in the FY2008 Consolidated Appropriations Act; P.L. 110-161) amends the Richard B. Russell National School Lunch Act to carry out these proposals.

Finally, a new issue arose during the farm bill debate in 2008, but has not yet been addressed in proposed or enacted legislation. Food assistance program benefits, whether they be meal subsidies for child nutrition programs or food stamp benefits, are indexed annually for food price inflation. However, with food prices rising rapidly, some argue that the existing annual indexing rule does not keep pace with the costs that schools and food stamp recipients face. This has led to calls for changes in food assistance program inflation indexing rules to more quickly reflect food price changes (although no legislation has yet been introduced).

PROPOSED LEGISLATION

As discussed earlier, the Administration announced its nutrition program (and other) proposals for the farm bill early in 2007 and included a few of them in its FY2008 appropriations request for food stamps. These were not formally introduced in legislative form; however as noted below, several bills include food stamp amendments close to some of the Administration's proposals. In addition, the House and Senate farm bills and the enacted farm bill (discussed later) include a few of its recommendations.

To date, the federal nutrition-assistance-related bills listed below have been introduced.

[Note: *Provisions in the following bills that are addressed (although not necessarily in the same way) in either the House, Senate, or enacted versions of the farm bill are italicized.*]

H.R. 45, Healthy Foods for Healthy Living Act

Authorizes grants to community-based organizations and other local agencies to promote greater consumption of fresh fruits, vegetables, and other healthy foods in low-income communities. Also covers services related to obesity prevention and treatment under Medicare and Medicaid.

H.R. 206, Anti-Hunger Empowerment Act of 2007

Raises federal cost sharing for state administrative expenses related to new activities increasing access to food stamps, requires reports on steps to improve access, and authorizes a pilot project providing "Beyond the Soup Kitchen" *grants to community-based groups for activities bolstering food security and technical assistance grants to community-based nonprofit feeding and anti-hunger groups*.

H.R. 208

Expands the existing free fresh fruit and vegetable program in schools to include schools in New York state and selected Head Start programs in participating states.

H.R. 1344

- *Increases and indexes required administrative funding for the Food* Distribution Program on Indian Reservations (FDPIR).
- *Requires and funds periodic surveys of the types of foods purchased* by schools with federal cash assistance for school meals.
- *Provides mandatory funding for a currently authorized pilot project* for raising the income limit for free school meals to 185% of the federal poverty income guidelines.

H.R. 1551 and S. 919, Healthy Farms, Fuels, and Foods Act of 2007

Title III — Healthy Food Choices

- Raises *the dollar amount for Community Food Projects, increases* federal matching, and expands the purposes of project grants.
- Expands the free fresh fruit and vegetable program in schools to *include at least 100 schools in every state and increase required* funding to $300 million a year.

Note: *Italicized provisions* in proposed legislation are those that have been addressed (although not necessarily in the same way) in the House, Senate, or enacted versions of the farm bill.

- Specifies an appropriations authorization of $20 million a year for grants to encourage schools' access to locally produced food (e.g., "farm-to-cafeteria" projects).
- Provides mandatory funding for the WIC Farmers' Market Nutrition program.
- Increases mandatory funding for the Senior Farmers' Market Nutrition program.
- Provides mandatory funding for the farmers' market promotion program — with money set aside to support the use of food stamp electronic benefit transfer systems in farmers' markets).
- Overrides current rules that limit the extent to which schools and other nutrition providers can specify a geographic preference (e.g., for locally produced food) when procuring food for the meals they serve.
- *Establishes a fruit and vegetable promotion program of matching grant assistance to trade organizations.*
- *Requires that foods and meals served in schools participating in* federal school meal programs meet the most recent Dietary Guidelines for Americans.
- *Increases the minimum requirement for specialty crop (e.g., fruit and vegetable) purchases using Section 32 funds to $400 million a year (from $200 million) and* raises the set-aside for fresh fruit and vegetable purchases through the DOD Fresh Program.
- *Defines "nutrition education" for purposes of funding under the Food Stamp Act (more broadly than under current rules) and* makes specific in food stamp law that nutrition education expenses are eligible for federal matching funding.
- Authorizes a pilot project under which food stamp recipients would receive financial incentives for the purchase of fresh fruit and vegetables.

H.R. 1600, EAT Healthy America Act

Title V — Nutrition

- *Expands the free fresh fruit and vegetable program in schools* to include at least 100 schools in every state and increases required funding to $300 million a year.
- Establishes a fruit and vegetable promotion program of matching grant assistance to trade organizations.

- Requires that foods and meals served in schools participating in federal school meal programs meet the most recent Dietary Guidelines for Americans.
- Increases the minimum requirement for specialty crop (e.g., fruit and vegetable) purchases using Section 32 funds to $400 million a year (from $200 million) and raises the set-aside for fresh fruit and vegetable purchases through the DOD Fresh program.
- Requires a study of school preferences as to the commodities supplied to them by the Agriculture Department, including the extent to which they prefer these commodities to include fresh fruit and vegetables, an analysis of logistical problems that impede distribution of fresh fruit and vegetables, and recommendations for improving the availability of fresh fruit and vegetables to schools.
- Requires an independent evaluation of the Agriculture Department's commodity purchasing processes, especially with regard to purchases of perishable specialty crops.
- Defines "nutrition education" for purposes of funding under the Food Stamp Act (more broadly than under current rules) and *makes specific in food stamp law that nutrition education expenses are eligible for federal matching funding.*
- Includes a sense of Congress provision stating that food stamp benefits should not be available to purchase nutrition supplements or anything other than food.
- Authorizes a pilot project under which food stamp recipients would receive financial incentives for the purchase of fresh fruit and vegetables.
- Requires decennial evaluations of WIC program food packages in light of the most recent Dietary Guidelines for Americans.
- Provides mandatory funding for the WIC Farmers' Market Nutrition program.
- Increases mandatory funding for the Senior Farmers' Market Nutrition program.

H.R. 2129, Feeding America's Families Act of 2007

Food Stamps

- Increases food stamp benefits for all eligible households over time by (1) raising basic (maximum) food stamp benefits to 103% of the inflation-adjusted cost of the Agriculture Department's "Thrifty Food Plan" (currently, benefits are set at 100% of the inflation- adjusted cost of this plan) and (2) *increasing and inflation indexing the minimum amount of household monthly income (the "standard deduction") that is disregarded when calculating benefits.*
- Increases food stamp benefits for households with dependent or child care expenses by removing dollar limits on the degree to which these costs are taken into account when calculating food stamp benefits (as in the Administration's proposal).
- Places into permanent law a rule that disregards combat-related pay for families with military members when calculating food stamp eligibility and benefits (as in the Administration's proposal).
- Increases the food stamp minimum monthly benefit.
- Increases the degree to which liquid assets are disregarded when judging food stamp eligibility by (1) increasing, and then indexing, the dollar limit on disregarded assets,

(2) requiring the disregard of all retirement savings (as in the Administration's proposal), and (3) requiring the disregard of savings for education (as in the Administration's proposal).

- Repeals the provisions of law substantially limiting food stamp participation by able-bodied adults without dependents (ABAWDs) who are not working at least half-time or in a work or training program.
- Makes all legally resident noncitizens eligible (if they meet other food stamp eligibility requirements), requires that state food stamp agencies not require "unnecessary" information from noncitizens who may be exempt from rules governing the attribution of financial resources from noncitizens' sponsors, and eases reporting requirements on state agencies in cases where they grant "indigence" exemptions from the rules for attribution of sponsors' financial resources.
- Requires states to "opt in" to rules limiting food stamp participation by convicted felons (as opposed to current provisions barring their receipt of food stamps unless a state "opts out").
- *Eases reporting requirements on elderly households* and allows state food stamp agencies to choose whether and how to act on information received through another program (unless it clearly indicates the household is not eligible for food stamps).
- Limits state food stamp agencies' ability to establish requirements as to how and when households receive their food stamp benefits.
- Limits state food stamp agencies' ability to delegate administrative responsibilities to non-state employees or entities and specifies the Agriculture Department's authority to limit contracting out these responsibilities.
- Increases required funding for grants to improve access to the Food Stamp program and simplify application for the program.
- Provides new funding for state agency initiatives to improve program access, efficiency, or integrity and requires funding for research or demonstration projects (primarily for studying ways to increase program access, reduce state agency and household administrative burdens, and improve program integrity).
- Increases required bonus payments to states achieving exemplary administrative performance.
- Increases federal matching payments for states' food stamp administrative costs in cases of natural disasters.
- Provides mandatory funding for grants to expand the number of farmers' markets that accept food stamp benefits in the form of EBT cards (e.g., providing equipment and training).

Other Provisions

- Indexes the $5 million a year provided for Community Food Projects funded under the Food Stamp Act.
- Increases required funding for commodities provided under The Emergency Food Assistance Program (TEFAP) from $140 million to $250 million in FY2008 — indexed in future years.

- Provides for funding of grants to support the work of food banks and similar nonprofit emergency feeding organizations in reducing hunger or food insecurity in their communities through improved infrastructure and obtaining, handling, storing, and distributing locally produced food.
- Provides funding to support grants to facilitate the procurement and transportation of highly perishable healthy food for low-income persons.
- Provides for funding of matching grants to organizations (like public food service providers, nonprofit organizations, and emergency feeding organizations) demonstrating that they have collaborated (or will collaborate) with local partner organizations in order to reduce hunger in communities that are underserved by existing programs or have high rates of food insecurity, hunger, poverty, or unemployment.
- Revamps provisions governing the Bill Emerson and Mickey Leland Hunger Fellowship program, particularly by providing mandatory funding.

H.R. 2144, Farm, Nutrition, and Community Investment Act of 2007

Title IV — Healthy Diets

- *Expands the free fresh fruit and vegetable program in schools* to include at least 100 schools in every state and increase required funding to $300 million a year.
- Increases the minimum requirement for specialty crop (e.g., fruit and vegetable) purchases using Section 32 funds to $400 million a year (from $200 million) and *raises the set-aside for fresh fruit and vegetable purchases through the DOD Fresh program.*
- Requires a study of school preferences as to the commodities supplied to them by the Agriculture Department, including the extent to which they prefer these commodities to include fresh fruit and vegetables, an analysis of logistical problems that impede distribution of fresh fruit and vegetables, and recommendations for improving the availability of fresh fruit and vegetables to schools.
- Requires an independent evaluation of the Agriculture Department's commodity purchasing processes, especially with regard to purchases of perishable specialty crops.
- Overrides current rules that limit the extent to which schools and farm-to-school programs can specify a geographic preference (e.g., for locally produced food) when procuring food for the meals they serve.
- Specifies an appropriations authorization of $20 million a year for grants to encourage schools' access to locally produced food (e.g., "farm-to-cafeteria" projects).
- Provides mandatory funding for the WIC Farmers' Market Nutrition program.
- Increases mandatory funding for the Senior Farmers' Market Nutrition program.
- Provides mandatory funding for pilot program to expand disabled individuals' access to farmers' markets.
- Provides mandatory funding for the farmers' market promotion program, with money set aside to support the use of food stamp electronic benefit transfer systems in farmers' markets.
- Title VI — Food Stamp Program and Other Nutrition Programs

- Bars any reductions in basic (maximum) food stamp benefit levels.
- Increases food stamp benefits for eligible households over time by increasing and inflation indexing the minimum amount of household monthly income (the "standard deduction") that is disregarded when calculating benefits.
- Increases food stamp benefits for households with dependent or child care expenses by removing dollar limits on the degree to which these costs are taken into account when calculating food stamp benefits (as in the Administration's proposal).
- Places into permanent law a rule that disregards combat-related pay for families with military members when calculating food stamp eligibility and benefits (as in the Administration's proposal).
- Increases the degree to which liquid assets are disregarded when judging food stamp eligibility by (1) increasing, and then indexing, the dollar limit on disregarded assets and (2) requiring the disregard of all retirement savings (as in the Administration's proposal).
- Eases reporting requirements on elderly households and allows state food stamp agencies to choose whether and how to act on information received through another program (unless it clearly indicates the household is not eligible for food stamps).
- Repeals the provisions of law substantially limiting food stamp participation by able-bodied adults without dependents (ABAWDs) who are not working at least half-time or in a work or training program.
- Increases the food stamp minimum monthly benefit.
- Limits states' ability to add eligibility requirements for food stamps (like biometric identification requirements).
- Limits states' ability to deny food stamp applications based on lack of verification.
- Substantially limits states' ability to delegate administrative responsibilities to non-state employees or entities.
- Makes all legally resident noncitizens eligible for food stamps (if they meet other eligibility requirements).
- Increases required funding for commodities provided under The Emergency Food Assistance Program (TEFAP) from $140 million to $250 million in FY2008 — indexed in future years.
- Raises the required amount for Community Food Projects, increases federal matching, and expands the purposes of project grants.

H.R. 2364, Local Food and Farm Support Act

- Provides mandatory funding for the WIC Farmers' Market Nutrition program.
- Increases mandatory funding for the Senior Farmers' Market Nutrition program.
- Raises the required amount for Community Food Projects, increases federal matching, and expands the purposes of project grants.
- Specifies an appropriations authorization of $20 million a year for grants to encourage schools' access to locally produced food (e.g., "farm-to-cafeteria" projects).

- Overrides current rules that limit the extent to which schools and farm-to-school programs can specify a geographic preference (e.g., for locally produced food) when procuring food for the meals they serve.
- Requires a study of school preferences as to the commodities supplied to them by the Agriculture Department, including the extent to which they prefer these commodities to include fresh fruit and vegetables, an analysis of logistical problems that impede distribution of fresh fruit and vegetables, and recommendations for improving the availability of fresh fruit and vegetables to schools.
- Establishes a demonstration project within the Food Stamp program under which recipients would receive financial incentives for increased purchases of fruits and vegetables.
- Requires an independent evaluation of the Agriculture Department's commodity purchasing processes, especially with regard to purchases of perishable specialty crops.

H.R. 2392, Family and Workplace Balancing Act of 2007

- In place of the current School Breakfast program, authorizes a school breakfast program in which free breakfasts are served to all children (without regard to family income).
- Requires the Department of Agriculture to establish a competitive grant program for local educational agencies to create healthy school nutrition environments and assess the effect of these environments on the health and well-being of their students. Provides mandatory funding of $10 million, rising to $35 million a year.
- Allows regulations that govern the service of any food in schools participating in federally subsidized school meal programs in competition with regular meal services. These regulations would apply to all school grounds during the school day, would not supersede state and local rules on competitive foods that conform to the nutritional goals of the regulations, require that all proceeds from any sale of competitive foods be used for the benefit of schools or student organizations, take into account differing needs of elementary, middle, and high schools, and implement required recommendations from the National Academy of Sciences' Institute of Medicine.
- Expands the provision of federal child nutrition subsidies for dinners served in after-school programs to all states.

H.R. 2401, Nutrition and Opportunities for the Underserved and Rural Incentives to Secure the Heartland (NOURISH) Act of 2007

Title VI — Healthy Food Choices

- Raises the required amount for Community Food Projects, increases federal matching, and expands the purposes of project grants.
- Expands the free fresh fruit and vegetable program in schools to include at least 100 schools in every state, increases required funding to $300 million a year.
- Specifies an appropriations authorization of $20 million a year for grants to encourage schools' access to locally produced food (e.g., "farm-to-cafeteria" projects).

- Provides mandatory funding for the WIC Farmers' Market Nutrition program.
- Increases mandatory funding for the Senior Farmers' Market Nutrition program.
- Provides mandatory funding for the farmers' market promotion program, with money set aside to support the use of food stamp electronic benefit transfer systems in farmers' markets.
- Overrides current rules that limit the extent to which schools and other nutrition providers can specify a geographic preference (e.g., *for locally produced food) when procuring food for the meals they serve.*
- Establishes a fruit and vegetable promotion program of matching grant assistance to trade organizations.
- Requires that foods and meals served in schools participating in federal school meal programs meet the most recent Dietary Guidelines for Americans.
- Increases the minimum requirement for specialty crop (e.g., fruit and vegetable) purchases using Section 32 funds to $400 million a year (from $200 million) and *raises the set-aside for fresh fruit and vegetable purchases through the DOD Fresh program.*
- Makes specific in food stamp law that nutrition education expenses are eligible for federal matching funding.
- Title IX — Nutrition
- *Renames the Food Stamp program* as the Secure Nutrition Access program.
- Increases food stamp benefits by increasing and inflation indexing the minimum amount of household monthly income (the "standard deduction") that is disregarded when calculating benefits.
- Increases food stamp benefits for households with dependent or child care expenses by removing dollar limits on the degree to which these costs are taken into account when calculating food stamp benefits (as in the Administration's proposal).
- Places into permanent law a rule that disregards combat-related pay for families with military members when calculating food stamp eligibility and benefits (as in the Administration's proposal).
- Increases, in steps, the food stamp minimum monthly benefit.
- Increases the degree to which liquid assets are disregarded when judging food stamp eligibility by (1) increasing, and then indexing, the dollar limit on disregarded assets, (2) requiring the disregard of all retirement savings (as in the Administration's proposal), and (3) requiring the disregard of savings for education (as in the Administration's proposal).
- Substantially loosens the provisions of law limiting food stamp participation by able-bodied adults without dependents (ABAWDs) who are not working at least half-time or in a work or training program.
- Makes all legally resident noncitizens eligible (if they meet other food stamp eligibility requirements), requires that state food stamp agencies not require "unnecessary" information from noncitizens who may be exempt from rules governing the attribution of financial resources from noncitizens' sponsors, and eases reporting requirements on state agencies in cases where they grant "indigence" exemptions from the rules for attribution of sponsors' financial resources.

- *Eases reporting requirements on elderly households* and allows state food stamp agencies to choose whether and how to act on information received through another program (unless it clearly indicates the household is not eligible for food stamps).
- Allows state agencies the option to allow "telephonic signatures" (recorded verbal consent) in applying for food stamps.
- Limits state food stamp agencies' ability to establish requirements as to how and when households receive their food stamp benefits.
- Limits state food stamp agencies' ability to delegate administrative responsibilities to non-state employees or entities and specifies the Agriculture Department's authority to limit contracting out these responsibilities.
- Increases required funding for grants to improve access to the Food Stamp program and simplify application for the program.
- Requires funding for research or demonstration projects (primarily for studying ways to increase program access, reduce state agency and household administrative burdens, and improve program integrity).
- Increases required bonus payments to states achieving exemplary administrative performance.
- Increases federal match payments for states' food stamp administrative costs in cases of natural disasters.
- Increases Puerto Rico's nutrition assistance grant and then indexes it for both food costs and population growth; *requires a study of the feasibility and effects of treating Puerto Rico as a state under the Food Stamp program.*
- Provides mandatory funding for grants to expand the number of farmers' markets that accept food stamp benefits in the form of EBT cards (e.g., providing equipment and training).
- Increases required funding for commodities provided under The Emergency Food Assistance Program (TEFAP) from $140 million to $250 million in FY2008, indexed in future years.

H.R. 2419, Farm, Nutrition, and Bioenergy Act of 2007

As approved by the House on July 27, 2007, includes substantial amendments affecting nutrition programs (Title IV). Senate version (the Food and Energy Security Act of 2007) was approved on December 14,2007. See the discussion of *Congressional Action* at the end of this report.

H.R. 2667, Disabled Farmers' Market Nutrition Pilot Program of 2007

Provides mandatory funding for pilot program to expand disabled individuals' access to farmers' markets.

H.R. 2720, Food and Agriculture Risk Management for the 21st Century Act of 2007 (FARM21 Act of 2007)

Title IIB — Healthy Foods

- Substantially increases funding for the program providing free fresh fruits and vegetables in schools and expands coverage of the program to all states.
- Specifies annual appropriations authorizations for grants to encourage schools' access to locally produced food (e.g., "farm-tocafeteria" projects).
- Provides mandatory funding for the farmers' market promotion program, with money set aside to *support the use of food stamp electronic benefit transfer systems in farmers' markets.*
- Establishes (and provides mandatory funding for) a fruit and vegetable promotion program of matching grant assistance to trade organizations.

Title IIF — Nutrition

- Places into permanent law a rule that disregards combat-related pay for families with military members when calculating food stamp eligibility and benefits (as in the Administration's proposal).
- Increases food stamp benefits for eligible households by increasing and inflation indexing the minimum amount of household monthly income (the "standard deduction") that is disregarded when calculating benefits.
- Increases food stamp benefits for households with dependent or child care expenses by removing dollar limits on the degree to which these costs are taken into account when calculating food stamp benefits (as in the Administration's proposal).
- Increases the food stamp minimum monthly benefit.
- Increases the degree to which liquid assets are disregarded when judging food stamp eligibility by requiring the disregard of all retirement savings (as in the Administration's proposal).
- *Eases reporting requirements on elderly* households and allows state food stamp agencies to choose whether and how to act on information received through another program (unless it clearly indicates the household is not eligible for food stamps).
- Increases required funding for grants to improve access to the Food Stamp program and simplify application for the program.
- Provides limited new funding for state initiatives to improve Food Stamp program access, efficiency, and integrity.
- Increases federal matching payments for states' food stamp administrative costs in cases of natural disasters.
- Increases funding for Community Food Projects.
- Provides funding for grants to expand the use of food stamp benefits through farmers' markets.
- Substantially increases mandatory funding for TEFAP commodities.
- Authorizes funding for a competitive grant program for emergency feeding organizations — to make infrastructure improvements and assist them in obtaining locally produced food.
- Authorizes funding to support grants to facilitate the procurement and transportation of highly perishable healthy food for low-income persons.

H.R. 3030, Summer Food Service Improvement Act of 2007

- Makes simplified summer food service program rules nationally applicable (see S. 790/H.R. 1740).
- Expands the summer food service program by increasing the number of areas in which free summer meals may be offered.
- Provides funding for start-up grants for new summer program sponsors.

H.R. 4000

Allows food stamp eligibility for citizens of the Freely Associated States of Micronesia, the Marshall Islands, and Palau who are resident in the United States.

S. 100, Healthy Students Act of 2007[31]

- Requires development of new nutritional standards for child nutrition programs and provides added funding to cover compliance with these standards in the Summer Food Service program.
- Authorizes a pilot project of grants to schools and nonprofit organizations to promote healthy nutrition alternatives through provision of organic foods, promotion of "healthy food education," operation of "farm-to-cafeteria" projects, and provision of professional development for teachers.

S. 541, Rural Opportunities Act of 2007

Overrides current rules that limit the extent to which schools and farm-to-school programs can specify a geographic preference (e.g., for locally produced food) when procuring food for the meals they serve.

S. 591, Food Stamp Personal Savings and Investment Act of 2007

Increases the degree to which liquid assets are disregarded when judging food stamp eligibility by (1) indexing the dollar limit on disregarded assets, (2) requiring the disregard of all retirement savings (as in the Administration's proposal), and (3) requiring the disregard of savings for education (as in the Administration's proposal).

S. 770, Food Stamp Vitamin and Mineral Improvement Act of 2007

Allows food stamp benefits to be used to purchase nutritional supplements.

S. 771/ H.R. 1363, Child Nutrition Promotion and School Lunch Protection Act of 2007

- Requires new regulations revising and expanding the definition of "food of minimal nutritional value" to be applied in schools participating in federally subsidized school meal programs.
- The new definition would effectively bar selling these foods outside school meal programs on school campuses at any time during the school day.
- The revised definition would take into account (1) the contributions of nutrients, ingredients, and foods to children's diets, (2) evidence concerning the relationship

between consumption of specific nutrients, ingredients, and foods in preventing and promoting the development of overweight, obesity, and chronic illnesses, (3) recommendations made by scientific organizations, and (4) special exemptions for school-sponsored fundraisers.

S. 790/H.R. 1740

Makes simplified summer food service program rules nationally applicable. These rules are intended to encourage expansion of the summer program by freeing summer program sponsors from a requirement that they provide detailed documentation of their expenses.

S. 1031, School Food Fresh Act of 2007

- Requires the establishment of a multi-agency USDA task force to evaluate, monitor, and provide coordination and direction for the Department's programs acquiring and distributing commodities to recipient agencies like schools, Indian reservations, and emergency feeding organizations. The task force is to review and make recommendations as to the specifications used for procuring commodities, their effective distribution, the best use of federal funds, and updates of the Dietary Guidelines for Americans.
- Authorizes competitive grants for evaluating commodity specifications.
- In place of the current set-aside of $50 million a year in funding for the DOD Fresh program for purchasing fresh fruits and vegetables for schools, effectively requires the Department of Agriculture to establish its own program for acquiring fruits and vegetables for schools (funded at the same level) and allows schools to divert up to 30% of their commodity "allowance" to purchase fruits and vegetables through the Department's program.
- Requires the Department of Agriculture to purchase commodities for distribution to schools and other outlets that are in the "least- processed state."

S. 1090, Senior Nutrition Act of 2007

Increases the income eligibility limit for elderly persons in the Commodity Supplemental Food Program (CSFP) from 130% to 185% of the federal poverty income guidelines.

S. 1160, Specialty Crop Competition Act of 2007

Title VI — Nutrition

- Increases the minimum requirement for specialty crop (e.g., fruit and vegetable) purchases using Section 32 funds to the amount spent in FY2001 plus $200 million a year and *raises the set-aside for fresh fruit and vegetable purchases through the DOD Fresh program.*
- *Expands the free fresh fruit and vegetable program* to all states and an additional 12 Indian reservations and increases mandatory funding.

- Defines "nutrition education" for purposes of funding under the Food Stamp Act (more broadly than under current rules) and *makes specific in food stamp law that nutrition education expenses are eligible for federal matching funding.*
- Authorizes a pilot project under which food stamp recipients would receive financial incentives for the purchase of fresh fruit and vegetables.
- Requires the Agriculture, Health and Human Services, and Education Departments to coordinate in establishing a Nutritional Education Program Review Committee. The Committee would submit a report describing methods of (1) evaluating the effectiveness of federal efforts to inform schools and other interested parties about federally-funded nutrition education programs, (2) improving these programs, and (3) making federal nutrition education funds more widely available.
- Includes a sense of the Senate provision stating that the Agriculture Department has an important role in educating families about nutrition and healthy lifestyles and that all federal nutrition programs should follow the latest nutritional science and be sensitive to the diverse cultures of the people they serve.

S. 1172, Hunger-Free Communities Act of 2007[32]

- Requires a study (with periodic updates) of matters relating to the problem of hunger in the United States and recommendations for removing obstacles to achieving a substantial reduction in domestic hunger. Domestic hunger goals are set at (1) a reduction of hunger to at or below 2% by 2010 and (2) a reduction in food insecurity to at or below 6% by 2010.
- Authorizes a program of matching grants to organizations (like public food service program providers, nonprofit organizations, and emergency feeding organizations) demonstrating that they have collaborated (or will collaborate) with local partner organizations in order to assess and reduce hunger in communities that are underserved by existing programs or have high rates of food insecurity, hunger, poverty, or unemployment.
- Authorizes a program of matching grants to emergency feeding organizations to support their infrastructure expansion activities and obtaining locally produced foods and wild game.
- Authorizes a program of matching grants to national or regional nonprofit organizations to provide training and technical assistance to help achieve domestic hunger reduction goals.
- Appropriations are authorized at $50 million a year.

S. 1422/H.R. 2720, Farm Risk Management Act for the 21st Century

Title IV — Nutrition Programs

- Places into permanent law a rule that disregards combat-related pay for families with military members when calculating food stamp eligibility and benefits (as in the Administration's proposal).

- Increases food stamp benefits by increasing and inflation indexing the minimum amount of household monthly income (the "standard deduction") that is disregarded when calculating benefits.
- Increases food stamp benefits for households with dependent or child care expenses by removing dollar limits on the degree to which these costs are taken into account when calculating food stamp benefits (as in the Administration's proposal).
- Increases the degree to which liquid assets are disregarded when judging food stamp eligibility by (1) requiring the disregard of all retirement savings (as in the Administration's proposal) and (2) requiring the disregard of savings for education (as in the Administration's proposal).
- Increases federal matching payments for states' food stamp administrative costs in cases of natural disasters — from the normal 50% to 90%.
- *Eases reporting requirements on elderly households* and allows state food stamp agencies to choose whether and how to act on information received through another program (unless it clearly indicates the household is not eligible for food stamps).
- Increases, in steps, the food stamp minimum monthly benefit.
- Increases required funding for grants to improve access to the Food Stamp program and simplify application for the program from $5 million to $15 million a year (indexed).
- Provides funding (up to $10 million a year in increased federal administrative matching money) for state initiatives to improve program access, efficiency, or integrity.
- Provides funding for projects to expand the number of farmers' markets that accept food stamps (through equipment, training, and technical assistance).
- Increases, in steps, funding for commodities provided by TEFAP — to $245 million in FY2011 — and indexes the amount for later years.
- Authorizes a program of competitive grants to emergency feeding organizations to support their infrastructure expansion activities and obtaining locally produced foods.
- Makes simplified summer food service program rules nationally applicable. These rules are intended to encourage expansion of the summer program by freeing summer program sponsors from a requirement that they provide detailed documentation of their expenses.
- Provides additional mandatory funding for expansion of the free fresh fruit and vegetable program in schools.
- Specifies an appropriations authorization for grants to encourage schools' access to locally produced food (e.g., "farm-to-cafeteria" projects) — $5 million a year rising to $10 million in FY201 1.
- Authorizes funding to support grants to facilitate the procurement and transportation of highly perishable healthy food for low-income persons.

S. 1424, Farm, Nutrition, and Community Investment Act of 2007

Title IV — Nutrition Programs

- Bars any reduction in basic (maximum) food stamp benefits based on the Agriculture Department's "Thrifty Food Plan."

- Places into permanent law a rule that disregards combat-related pay for families with military members when calculating food stamp eligibility and benefits (as in the Administration's proposal).
- Increases food stamp benefits by increasing and inflation indexing the minimum amount of household monthly income (the "standard deduction") that is disregarded when calculating benefits.
- Increases food stamp benefits for households with dependent or child care expenses by removing dollar limits on the degree to which these costs are taken into account when calculating food stamp benefits (as in the Administration's proposal).
- Increases the degree to which liquid assets are disregarded when judging food stamp eligibility by (1) indexing the dollar limit on disregarded assets and (2) requiring the disregard of all retirement savings (as in the Administration's proposal).
- *Eases reporting requirements on elderly households* and allows state food stamp agencies to choose whether and how to act on information received through another program (unless it clearly indicates the household is not eligible for food stamps).
- Repeals the provisions of law substantially limiting food stamp participation by able-bodied adults without dependents (ABAWDs) who are not working at least half-time or in a work or training program.
- Makes all legally resident noncitizens eligible (if they meet other food stamp eligibility requirements), requires that state food stamp agencies not require "unnecessary" information from noncitizens who may be exempt from rules governing the attribution of financial resources from noncitizens' sponsors, and eases reporting requirements on state agencies in cases where they grant "indigence" exemptions from the rules for attribution of sponsors' financial resources.
- Increases the food stamp minimum monthly benefit.
- Limits state food stamp agencies' ability to delegate administrative responsibilities to non-state employees or entities and requires that no food stamp application be denied for lack of verification unless the state agency determines that the applicant household has refused to comply with a request made by a state agency employee (e.g., not a contractor).
- Raises the required amount for Community Food Projects, increases federal matching, and expands the purposes of project grants.
- Increases required funding for commodities provided under The Emergency Food Assistance Program (TEFAP) from $140 million to $250 million in FY2008 — indexed in future years.
- Requires a study of the feasibility and effects of treating Puerto Rico as a state under the Food Stamp program.

Title VIII — Healthy Diets

- *Expands the free fresh fruit and vegetable program in schools* to include at least 100 schools in every state and increases required funding to $300 million a year.
- Specifies an appropriations authorization of $20 million a year for grants to encourage schools' access to locally produced food (e.g., "farm-to-cafeteria" projects).

- Increases the minimum requirement for specialty crop (e.g., fruit and vegetable) purchases using Section 32 funds to $400 million a year (from $200 million) and *raises the set-aside for fresh fruit and vegetable purchases through the DOD Fresh program.*
- Requires a study of school preferences as to the commodities supplied to them by the Department of Agriculture, including the extent to which they prefer these commodities to include fresh fruit and vegetables, an analysis of logistical problems that impede distribution of fresh fruit and vegetables, and recommendations for improving the availability of fresh fruit and vegetables to schools.
- Requires an independent evaluation of the Agriculture Department's commodity purchasing processes, especially with regard to purchases of perishable specialty crops.
- Provides mandatory funding for the WIC Farmers' Market Nutrition program.
- Increases mandatory funding for the Senior Farmers' Market Nutrition program.
- Overrides current rules that limit the extent to which schools and other nutrition providers can specify a geographic preference (e.g., for locally produced food) when procuring food for the meals they serve.

S. 1432, Food Outreach and Opportunity Development for a Healthy America Act of 2007

Title I — Food Stamp Program

- Raises funding for Community Food Projects.
- Defines "nutrition education" for purposes of funding under the Food Stamp Act (more broadly than under current rules) and sets aside at least $100 million a year for nutrition education.

Title II — National School Lunch Program

- *Expands the free fresh fruit and vegetable program in schools* to include at least 100 schools in every state and increases required funding to $300 million a year.
- Specifies an appropriations authorization of $20 million a year for grants to encourage schools' access to locally produced food (e.g., "farm-to-cafeteria" projects).
- Overrides current rules that limit the extent to which schools and other nutrition providers can specify a geographic preference (e.g., for locally produced food) when procuring food for the meals they serve.

Title IV — Miscellaneous

- Provides mandatory funding for the farmers' market promotion program at $25 million a year and expands the types of activities that may be supported.
- Provides mandatory funding for the Senior Farmers' Market Nutrition program.

S. 1529, Food Stamp Fairness and Benefit Restoration Act of 2007

Food Stamps

- Increases food stamp benefits by inflation indexing the minimum amount of household monthly income (the "standard deduction") that is disregarded when calculating benefits.
- Increases food stamp benefits for households with dependent or child care expenses by removing dollar limits on the degree to which these costs are taken into account when calculating food stamp benefits (as in the Administration's proposal).
- Increases the degree to which liquid assets are disregarded when judging food stamp eligibility by (1) indexing the dollar limit on disregarded assets, (2) requiring the disregard of all retirement savings (as in the Administration's proposal), and (3) requiring the disregard of savings for education (as in the Administration's proposal).
- Makes all legally resident noncitizens eligible (if they meet other food stamp eligibility requirements), requires that state food stamp agencies not require "unnecessary" information from noncitizens who may be exempt from rules governing the attribution of financial resources from noncitizens' sponsors, and eases reporting requirements on state agencies in cases where they grant "indigence" exemptions from the rules for attribution of sponsors' financial resources.
- Significantly loosens the provisions of law limiting food stamp participation by able-bodied adults without dependents (ABAWDs) who are not working at least half-time or in a work or training program.

The Emergency Food Assistance Program (TEFAP)

- Increases required funding for commodities provided under TEFAP from $140 million to $180 million a year.

S. 1575, Food Employment Empowerment and Development Program Act of 2007 (the FEED Act of 2007)

Authorizes grants to public agencies and private nonprofit organizations for the purposes of (1) recovering donated food from food service businesses (e.g., restaurants) and farms, (2) distributing meals or recovered food to entities feeding vulnerable populations, (3) training unemployed or underemployed adults in food service careers, and (4) carrying out "welfare-to-work" programs in combination with the production of school and after-school meal programs.

S. 1755/H.R. 2968, Summer Food Service Rural Expansion Act

Makes nationally applicable rules (now used in a pilot project in Pennsylvania) that ease participation by summer program sponsors in rural areas.

S. 2066, Back to School: Improving Standards for Nutrition and Physical Education in Schools Act of 2007

Requires that new, expanded regulations governing the offering of "foods of minimal nutritional value" in schools that are consistent with standards established by the National Academy of Sciences' Institute of Medicine. These standards would cover schools participating in federally subsidized school meal programs and be applied to all foods and beverages sold on school campuses at any time. Requires standards for physical activity in all schools receiving federal funds.

S. 2143/H.R. 3978, Student Breakfast and Education Improvement Act of 2007

Authorizes competitive grants to schools to help establish, promote, or expand school breakfast programs and for related purposes (e.g., to increase local or fresh foods available in school breakfast programs, extend breakfast periods, and increase participation in breakfast programs).

S. 2228, Farm, Ranch, Equity, Stewardship, and Health Act of 2007 (FRESH Act)

Title III, Subtitle C — Nutrition

- Increases funding for the fresh fruit and vegetable program — to $200 million a year.
- Specifies an appropriations authorization of $20 million a year for grants to encourage schools' access to locally produced food (e.g., "farm-to-cafeteria" projects).
- Provides mandatory funding for the WIC Farmers' Market Nutrition program.
- Provides mandatory funding for the Senior Farmers' Market Nutrition program and bars federal limits on benefit levels.
- Requires that foods and meals served in schools participating in federal school meal programs meet the most recent Dietary Guidelines for Americans.
- Authorizes a pilot project under which food stamp recipients would receive financial incentives for the purchase of fresh fruits and vegetables.
- Overrides current rules that limit the extent to which schools and the Defense Department can specify a geographic preference (e.g., for locally produced food) when procuring food for the meals they serve.
- Increases (and makes mandatory) funding for Community Food Projects, increases federal cost-sharing for the projects, and expands the purposes for which they may be used.
- Increases minimum required purchases of fruits and vegetables using Section 32 funds and expands the set-aside for DOD Fresh program purchases.

Title V — Nutrition; Subtitle A — Food Stamp Program

- Places into permanent law a rule that disregards combat-related military pay for families with military members when calculating food stamp eligibility and benefits (as in the Administration's proposal).
- Increases food stamp benefits by increasing (to $147) and inflation indexing the minimum amount of household monthly income (the "standard deduction") that is disregarded when calculating benefits.
- Increases food stamp benefits for households with dependent or child care expenses by removing dollar limits on the degree to which these costs are taken into account when calculating benefits (as in the Administration's proposal).
- Increases the degree to which liquid assets are disregarded when judging food stamp eligibility by (1) indexing the dollar limit on disregarded assets and (2) disregarding all

tax-recognized retirement savings and retirement savings plans and educational savings.

- Eases provisions of law limiting the eligibility of able-boded adults without dependents (ABAWDs) who are not working or in a work or training program.
- Increases funding for TEFAP commodities in FY2008 to $250 million.

Title V — Nutrition; Subtitle B — *Food Service Industry Job Training for Low-Income Adults*

- Authorizes a grant program for recovery of donated foods from food service businesses (e.g., restaurants) and farms, distribution of meals or the recovered foods to nonprofit organizations and those serving vulnerable populations (e.g., the homeless, at-risk youths), training of unemployed and underemployed adults for food service careers, and carrying out welfare-to-work job training programs linked to the provision of school meals or support of after-school programs (see S. 1575).
- Authorizes grants to food program service providers and local nonprofit organizations (like emergency feeding organizations) for projects that assess community hunger problems and meet, or develop new resources or programs to meet, goals for achieving hunger-free communities (see S. 1172).

Title V — Nutrition; Subtitle C — Other Programs

- Makes simplified summer food service program rules nationally applicable (see S. 790/H.R. 1740).
- Requires continuation of current nutrition status monitoring and related research activities by the Secretaries of Agriculture and Health and Human Services.

S. 2302, Food and Energy Security Act of 2007

As reported by the Senate Committee on Agriculture, Nutrition, and Forestry on November 2, 2007 (S.Rept. 110-220), includes substantial amendments affecting nutrition programs (Title IV). Adopted by the Senate, with substantial amendments, as its version of H.R. 2419, on December 14, 2007. See discussion of congressional action below.

S. 2726, Bonus TEFAP Assistance Act of 2008

Provides mandatory funding to states for transportation, storage, and distribution costs associated with "bonus" commodities donated through The Emergency Food Assistance Program (TEFAP).

S. 2745/H.R. 5578, P.L. 110-196 (enacted March 14, 2008)

Extends expired authorities for most programs covered by the nutrition title (and other titles) of the pending farm bill until April 18, 2008.

Congressional Action

In addition to making FY2008 Agriculture Department appropriations covering all the nutrition assistance programs (P.L. 110-161; 2008 Consolidated Appropriations Act), Congress has acted legislatively in four areas related to domestic food assistance.[33]

Older Americans Act Nutrition Programs

On April 23, 2007, P.L. 110-19 was enacted. This law makes clear that nutrition programs for the elderly operated under the authority of the Older Americans Act (home-delivered meals and congregate meal projects) may use their Older Americans Act funding to obtain food commodities through the Agriculture Department for meals they serve.

Simplified Summer Food Service Rules

As noted earlier in the discussion of other domestic food assistance issues and proposals, P.L. 110-161 includes an amendment to the Richard B. Russell National School Lunch Act that makes "simplified summer food service rules" applicable nationwide. These rules (allowed to be used in 26 states and Puerto Rico) are intended to encourage expansion of the Summer Food Service program by freeing project sponsors from a requirement that they provided detailed documentation of their expenses in order to receive standard program per-meal subsidy rates; this matches rules for the regular School Lunch program.[34]

Suppers in after-School Programs

As discussed earlier in the section on other domestic food aid issues and proposals, P.L. 110-161 incorporates an amendment to the Richard B. Russell National School Lunch Act that extends federal subsidies for suppers served in after- school programs to one additional state — West Virginia — bringing the total number of states in which this assistance is offered to eight.

Expiring Authorities[35]

At the end of FY2007 (and with no enacted farm bill to extend them), a number of authorities in domestic food assistance (and other farm-bill-related) laws expired. They were effectively extended by a series of appropriations actions, beginning with P.L. 110-161, the 2008 Consolidated Appropriations Act, and ending with P.L. 110- 231. These laws provided continued funding for all domestic food assistance programs and kept in force certain legislative authorities in domestic food assistance laws that also expired with FY2007.

2008 Farm Bill

House Bill Provisions

On June 15, 2007, the House Agriculture Committee's Subcommittee on Departmental Operations Oversight, Nutrition, and Forestry forwarded its recommendations for the nutrition title of the farm bill to the full committee. On July 19, 2007, the House Agriculture Committee approved its version of the farm bill (H.R. 2419; H.Rept. 110-256), accepting the subcommittee's proposals with minor amendments. On July 27, 2007, the House adopted H.R. 2419, with amendments.

The House bill's nutrition title (Title IV) incorporated the significant changes to law noted below. Most of the amendments in the House bill did not directly affect nutrition program costs. However, a number of important provisions did, and the required new funding (generally from tax law changes) was provided in the bill. The Congressional Budget Office estimate of the cost of the provisions of the nutrition title (using its March 2007 "baseline" assumptions) projected that they would add some $4.2 billion in federal spending (budget authority and outlays) over the next five years (the "life" of the farm bill).[36] Six provisions of Title IV accounted for virtually all of its cost in the first five years: increasing food stamp benefits by raising the "standard deduction" disregard of income (52%), boosting food stamp benefits by eliminating limits on income disregards tied to dependent care expenses (6%), raising minimum food stamp benefits (6%), increasing food stamp dollar limits on allowable liquid assets and disregarding retirement savings/plans and education savings as countable assets when judging food stamp eligibility (15%), increasing mandatory spending on TEFAP commodities (14%), and expanding support for the fresh fruit and vegetable program in schools (7%). As can be seen, the large majority of new spending generated in the House bill was tied to changes in food stamp law — that is, $3.3 billion over the next five years.

Over the next ten years, changes made by the House bill were expected to cost a total of $11.5 billion (using March 2007 "baseline" assumptions), because its revisions were made part of permanent law, unlike the Senate's measure.

Food Stamps

General Provisions

- Renamed the Food Stamp program the Secure Supplemental Nutrition Assistance program.
- Made coupons issued under the Food Stamp program — prior to the changeover to electronic benefit transfer (EBT) cards as the method of issuing benefits — no longer redeemable.

Benefit Levels and Eligibility [37]

- Increased benefits (and, to a limited degree, liberalized income eligibility standards) for most households by raising and then indexing the minimum amount of household monthly income (the "standard deduction") that is disregarded when calculating household benefits (and, to a limited degree, income eligibility). The monthly standard deduction was initially increased by 8%, from $134 to $145 a month, for an initial benefit increase of about $3-$4 a month for most households. This change accounted for just over half of the new spending brought on by the provisions of the nutrition title.

- Increased benefits (and, to a limited degree, liberalized income eligibility standards) for some households with dependent or child care expenses by removing the dollar limits on the degree to which these expenses are taken into account (i.e., disregarded in calculating household income).[38] This change accounted for about 6% of the new spending expected under the provisions of the nutrition title.
- Increased minimum benefits for recipient households near the income eligibility limits by calculating minimum benefits as 10% of the (indexed) maximum monthly benefit for a one-person household. The minimum benefit ($10 a month for one- and two-person households) would be initially lifted to an estimated $16 a month. This change represented some 6% of the new spending in the nutrition title.
- Placed into permanent law a rule (now in annual appropriations laws) that disregards combat-related pay for families with military members when calculating benefits (and, to a limited degree, income eligibility).[39]
- Adopted the Administration's proposal to bar food stamp eligibility to those disqualified from the FDPIR.

Asset Eligibility Standards

- Increased the degree to which liquid assets are disregarded when judging eligibility by annually indexing the dollar limits on assets an eligible household may hold.[40]
- Added to the list of assets that are to be disregarded all tax- recognized retirement savings/plans and education savings.[41] These changes, coupled with indexing the dollar limits on assets, accounted for about 15% of the new spending in the nutrition title.

Program Administration and Nutrition Education

- Substantially limited states' authority to "privatize" program administration (to delegate food stamp administrative responsibilities to non-government employees or entities) by restricting most communications with households and participation in determinations relating to compliance with substantive or procedural program requirements (or most other determinations) to government "merit system" employees. Denied federal matching funds where these limits are not observed.
- Adopted the Administration's proposals with regard to "widespread systemic errors" in states' administration of food stamps — allowing the Agriculture Department to effectively waive requirements to collect overissued benefits from recipients in the case of a major systemic administrative failure and to require states to repay overissued benefits in such cases.
- Loosened benefit "accrual" rules limiting how long recipients can leave their electronic benefit accounts inactive before their benefits are recovered.
- Placed into law specific rules governing the use of "telephonic signatures" for food stamp applications.
- Put into law existing policy allowing approval of faith-based organizations operating residential substance abuse treatment programs as eligible to receive food stamp benefits on behalf of their residents.

- Placed into law provisions comparable to pre-existing policies supporting (and providing federal 50% matching funds for) nutrition education for the food-stamp-eligible population. Called on the Agriculture Department to encourage and support the most effective interventions (including public health approaches as well as traditional education). Stated that food stamp program nutrition education activities should be coordinated with other federally funded food assistance and should leverage public/private partnerships.

Retailers

- Adopted the Administration's proposals with regard to penalties on retailers for violations of food stamp law/regulations — giving more authority to impose fines in lieu of disqualification for minor violations and new authority to fine retailers in addition to disqualification for major violations; allowed the Agriculture Department to suspend redemption of retailers' food stamp receipts pending disqualification in "certain egregious trafficking cases."[42]

Other Provisions and Programs

Reauthorization

- Extended all expiring authorities in the Food Stamp Act and other laws governing programs covered in the nutrition title (including authorizations for appropriations and mandatory spending directives) through FY2012. Amendments made in the House bill generally were made part of permanent law.

The Emergency Food Assistance Program (TEFAP)

- Increased mandatory funding for TEFAP commodities from $140 million to $250 million in FY2008, indexed for food price inflation in later years. This change accounted for about 14% of the new spending in the nutrition title.
- Boosted the authorized appropriations level for funding of TEFAP distribution costs from $60 million to $100 million a year.

Fruits and Vegetables

- Increased mandatory funding for the current program offering free fresh fruits and vegetables in elementary and secondary schools, from up to $15 million in mandatory and discretionary money available in FY2006 and FY2007, to $70 million a year (mandatory). This increase represented 7% of the new spending in the nutrition title.
- Expanded availability of this school fresh fruit and vegetable program to all states (from the current 14 states). At least 35 elementary and secondary schools in each state would participate, and additional schools would participate in accordance with the state's proportion of the student population.
- Allowed the Agriculture Department to reserve up to 1% of the school fresh fruit and vegetable program funding for administrative costs, and allowed states to reserve up to 5% for administrative expenses.

- Increased the minimum set-aside of mandatory funding to purchase fresh fruits and vegetables for child nutrition providers (e.g., schools) through the DOD Fresh Program, from $50 million a year to $75 million a year.

Commodity Supplemental Food Program (CSFP)

- Increased income eligibility limits for elderly applicants to the CSFP (from 130% to 185% of the federal poverty income guidelines, the same standard applied to households with women, infants, and children).

Community Food Projects

- Authorized funding for community food projects at $30 million a year, up from the existing set-aside of $5 million a year.
- Expanded the purposes for which community food project grants can be used to include initiatives related to (1) transportation and processing of local foods; (2) retail access to healthy food in underserved markets; (3) integration of urban- and metro-area food production into food projects; and (4) technical assistance for youth, socially disadvantaged individuals, and groups with limited resources.
- Increased the limit on the federal share of project grants from 50% to 75%.
- Raised the limit on the number of years for which grants may be awarded from three to five years.
- Increased the set-aside for a special grant for "innovative programs" from $200,000 to $500,000.

Food Distribution Program on Indian Reservations (FDPIR)

- Authorized funding ($5 million a year) for a fund to purchase traditional and locally grown food for the FDPIR, at least 50% of which must be produced by Native American farmers, ranchers, and producers.
- Required a report reviewing the procedures for determining FDPIR food packages and the adequacy of the food packages and describing any plans to revise the packages to conform with the most recent Dietary Guidelines for Americans.

Senior Farmers' Market Nutrition Program (SFMNP)

- Authorized additional appropriations to expand the SFMNP: $20 million for FY2008 rising, in stages, to $75 million for FY20 12.
- Adopted the Administration's proposals to disregard SFMNP benefits under welfare laws and bar sales taxes on them.

Geographic Preference and Buy American Rules

- Generally overrode rules that limit the extent to which schools and the DOD Fresh program can specify a geographic preference (e.g., for locally produced food items) when procuring food for meals served by child nutrition providers.
- Encouraged the Agriculture Department to undertake training, guidance, and enforcement to implement existing Buy American requirements for child nutrition programs.

Puerto Rico

- Directed a comprehensive study of extending the regular Food Stamp program to Puerto Rico as a state (in lieu of its nutrition assistance block grant).

Obesity Initiative

- Authorized appropriations ($10 million a year) for a competitive grant initiative to address obesity among low-income Americans, similar to the proposal advanced by the Administration.

Bill Emerson and Mickey Leland Hunger Fellowship Program

- Revamped provisions of law governing the Emerson-Leland Hunger Fellowship program.[43] Authorized appropriations of $3 million a year.

Nutrition Monitoring

- Required continuation of joint national nutrition monitoring activities — established under the 1990 Nutrition Monitoring and Related Research Act — by the Departments of Agriculture and Health and Human Services.

Sense of Congress: Juvenile Obesity

- Provides that it is the sense of Congress that food items in school meal programs should be selected so as to reduce the incidence of juvenile obesity and maximize nutritional value.

Senate Bill Provisions

On December 14, 2007, the Senate adopted its version of the farm bill, a substitute for H.R. 2419, based on S. 2302 (S.Rept. 110- 220) as amended on the Senate floor.

As passed, the Senate bill's nutrition title (Title IV) incorporated the significant changes to law noted below. As with the House bill, most of its amendments did not directly affect nutrition program costs. But a number of important provisions did, and the required offsetting funding — from savings in other (agriculture) programs and titles in the bill — was provided. Estimates from the Congressional Budget Office (using its March 2007 "baseline" assumptions) placed the overall five-year cost (new budget authority) at $5.4 billion, or $5.3 billion in new outlays.[44] Changes to the Food Stamp program and TEFAP and expansion of the fresh fruit and vegetable program in schools accounted for 97% of the new spending in the Senate bill. Food stamp amendments alone represented 66% of the new spending ($3.5 billion); the four most expensive of these revisions were an increase in the "standard deduction" disregard of income, loosened asset eligibility rules, a higher minimum monthly benefit, and removal of dollar limits on income disregards tied to dependent care expenses. New TEFAP spending accounted for 10% of the added spending ($550 million). And additional money for the fruit and vegetable program represented 21% ($1.1 billion). As can be seen, in a major difference from the House bill, the Senate's version placed substantially more emphasis on support for the fresh fruit and vegetable program, both in absolute dollar terms and as a proportion of total spending under the nutrition title.

In another large difference from the House bill, the Senate's measure was expected to cost only $5.6 billion over the next ten years (as opposed to the House's $11.5 billion), because most of its major revisions were terminated after FY20 12 (not made permanent) for budgetary reasons.

Food Stamps

General Provisions

- Renamed the Food Stamp program the *Food and Nutrition program.*
- Made coupons issued under the Food Stamp program — prior to the changeover to electronic benefit transfer (EBT) cards as the method of issuing benefits — no longer redeemable.

Benefit Levels and Eligibility[45]

- Increased benefits (and, to a limited degree, liberalized income eligibility standards) for most households by raising and then indexing the minimum amount of household monthly income (the "standard deduction") that is disregarded when calculating household benefits (and, to a limited degree, income eligibility). The monthly standard deduction would be initially increased by 4.5%, from $134 to $140 a month, for an initial benefit increase of about $2-$3 a month for most households. This change accounted for about one-quarter of the new spending brought on by the provisions of the nutrition title.
- Increased benefits (and, to a limited degree, liberalized income eligibility standards) for some households with dependent or child care expenses by removing the dollar limits on the degree to which these expenses are taken into account (i.e., disregarded in calculating household income).[46] This change was the same as in the House bill and accounted for about 4% of the new spending expected under the nutrition title.
- Increased minimum benefits for recipient households near the income eligibility limits by calculating minimum benefits as 10% of the (indexed) maximum monthly benefit for a one-person household. The minimum benefit ($10 a month for one- and two-person households) would initially rise to an estimated $16 a month. This revision was the same as in the House bill represented some 4% of the new spending under the nutrition title.
- Placed into permanent law a rule (now in annual appropriations laws) that disregards combat-related pay for families with military members when calculating benefits (and, to a limited degree, income eligibility).[47] This amendment was the same as in the House bill.
- As in the House bill, adopted the Administration's proposal to bar food stamp eligibility to those disqualified from the FDPIR.
- Lengthened the eligibility period for able-bodied adults without dependents (ABAWDs) who are not working or in a work/training program from 3 months in every 36-month period to 6 months in every 36-month period. Also eliminated a current provision under which ABAWDs who gain eligibility by meeting the work or work/training test, but subsequently fail to meet the test, may remain eligible for an additional 3 consecutive months.
- Allowed states to provide transitional food stamp benefits to households with children that cease to receive cash assistance under a state-funded public assistance

program, as is the case for households losing federally financed Temporary Assistance for Needy Families (TANF) benefits. Transitional benefits consist of five months' benefits based on the benefit immediately prior to losing cash assistance (and adjusted for the loss of cash aid).

- Similar to suggestions by the Administration, allowed disqualification of individuals found by a court or administrative agency to have intentionally (1) obtained cash by misusing program benefits to obtain money for return deposits on containers or (2) sold any food purchased with program benefits. (Also noted in *Retailers and Use of Benefits* below.)

Asset Eligibility Standards

- Increased the degree to which liquid assets are disregarded when judging eligibility by first increasing the dollar limits on assets an eligible household may hold and then annually indexing the new limits. The initial increase would be from $2,000 to $3,500 for most households and from $3,000 to $4,500 to households with elderly or disabled members.
- As in the House bill, adopted the Administration recommendation to add to the list of assets that are to be disregarded all tax-recognized retirement savings/plans and education savings. These changes, together with the increased and indexed dollar limits noted above, accounted for about one-quarter of the new spending in the Senate's nutrition title.

Program Administration and Nutrition Education

- Required standards for identifying major changes in state agency administrative operations, such as substantial increases in reliance on automated systems and potential increases in administrative burdens placed on applicants or recipients. Further mandated that, if a state agency implements a major change in operations, it must notify the Agriculture Department and collect any information the Department needs to identify and correct any adverse effects on program integrity or access.
- Required that computerized systems for state agency operations must (1) be tested adequately before and after implementation and (2) be operated under a plan for continuous updating and testing.
- As in the House bill, adopted the Administration recommendation with regard to "widespread systemic errors" in states' administration of food stamps — allowing the Agriculture Department to effectively waive requirements to collect overissued benefits from recipients in the case of major systemic administrative failure and to require states to repay overissued benefits in such cases.
- . Expanded the application of "simplified reporting" rules. Allowed states to extend periodic reporting of changes in household circumstances (as opposed to reporting all changes when they occur) to households with elderly or disabled members (and certain others). Limited the frequency with which these households must report (other than changes whereby they exceed the gross monthly income eligibility limits), for example, to no more often than once a year for elderly or disabled households with no earned income.

- Similar to the House bill, allowed households to accrue unused benefits under the electronic benefit transfer system for up to 12 month before they are expunged. Also required states to notify households of electronically stored (unused) benefits and make them available not later than 48 hours after a household's request.
- Required consistent federally established procedures for identifying felons fleeing from active pursuit for prosecution or custody; so- called "fleeing felons" are ineligible for food stamps.
- Required that any method for staggering issuance of benefits throughout a month not include splitting any household's benefit into multiple issuances.
- As in the House bill, placed into law specific rules governing the use of "telephonic signatures" for food stamp applications.
- Expanded privacy protections for applicants and recipients to control the release of information obtained from them to third parties.
- Allowed "job retention services" provide to those who have obtained employment to be treated as an employment and training program eligible for support for food stamp purposes.
- Allowed individuals who volunteer for employment and training programs for food stamp recipients to participate for more than the maximum 20 hours a week (or a number of hours based on their benefit and the minimum wage).
- Required states to analyze and demonstrate the cost-effectiveness of biometric identification technology (like fingerprinting) in order to receive a federal administrative share of the cost.
- Limited the time that unspent federal funding for the basic expenses of employment and training programs for food stamp recipients may remain available to two years and rescinded currently unspent employment and training money.
- Similar to the House bill, specified in law that states may implement nutrition education programs promoting healthy food choices for those eligible for food stamps and may receive federal 50% matching funds for these initiatives.

Retailers and Use of Benefits

- Similar to the House bill and the Administration's proposals, revised rules with regard to penalties on retailers for violations of food stamp law or regulations. Allowed fines of up to $100,000 per violation in all cases, including where a disqualification has been imposed (vs. up to $10,000 per violation as an alternative to disqualification). Removed minimum disqualification periods for first and second offenses. Eased conditions under which a bond may be required of a previously violating retailer who wishes to re-enter the program. Allowed the Agriculture Department to suspend retailers' payments for food stamp receipts pending disqualification in cases of flagrant violations.
- Disqualified benefit recipient misusing food stamps to obtain container deposits or by selling food purchased with program benefits (also noted in *Benefit Levels and Eligibility* above).
- Required regulations defining dietary supplements and provided that no dietary supplements may be purchased with program benefits until final regulations have been issued or a voluntary system of labeling for identification of eligible dietary supplements has been certified.

Other Provisions and Programs

Reauthorization

- Extended all significant expiring authorities in the Food Stamp Act and other laws governing programs covered in the nutrition title (including authorizations of appropriations and mandatory spending directives) indefinitely — with the exception of the authorization of funding for community food projects (extended through FY20 12). Amendments made by the Senate bill generally terminated with FY2012.

The Emergency Food Assistance Program (TEFAP)

- Increased mandatory funding for TEFAP commodities from $140 million to $250 million a year, beginning with FY2008. This change accounted for about 10% of the new spending in the nutrition title.
- As in the House bill, boosted the authorized appropriations level for funding of TEFAP distribution costs from $60 million to $100 million a year.
- Required that state TEFAP plans of operation be submitted every three years instead of every four years.
- Specifically allowed the use of funding provided for TEFAP processing, storage, and other distribution expenses for costs related to donated wild game.

Fruits and Vegetables

- Replaced the pre-existing program offering free fresh fruits and vegetables in elementary and secondary schools, beginning with the 2008-2009 school year. Provided mandatory funding of $225 million (FY2008) annually, indexed for inflation, for a new program that would be available in a limited number of state-selected elementary schools nationwide, including at least 100 schools on Indian reservations. Funds would be allocated among states in two tranches: a minimum grant for each state and an amount based on state population. Per-student grants would be between $50 and $75, annually, and set by states. An evaluation would be required by 2011. This program represented 21% of the new spending in the nutrition title.

Commodity Supplemental Food Program (CSFP)

- Prohibited federal requirements as to giving priority to either (1) elderly or (2) women, infants, and children in CSFP projects.
- Permitted states to serve elderly persons with income up to 185% of the federal poverty guidelines, if the Secretary determines that annual appropriations have enabled every state wishing to participate in the CSFP to do so.

Community Food Projects

- Increased maximum funding for community food projects from $5 to $10 million a year (through FY20 12).

Food Distribution Program on Indian Reservations (FDPIR)

- Similar to the House bill, authorized $5 million a year for a fund to purchase "traditional" and local foods for the FDPIR.

- As in the House bill, required a report reviewing the procedures for determining FDPIR food packages and the adequacy of the packages and describing any plans to revise the packages to conform with the most recent Dietary Guidelines for Americans.
- Specifically permitted the Agriculture Department to purchase, subject to appropriations, bison meat for distribution through the FDPIR, including meat from Native American producers and producer-owned cooperatives.

Senior Farmers' Market Nutrition Program (SFMNP)

- Increased mandatory funding for the SFMNP from $15 million to $25 million a year.
- As in the House bill, adopted the Administration's proposals to disregard SFMNP benefits under welfare laws and bar sales taxes on them.

Farmers' Markets and EBT Cards

- Provided mandatory funding ($5 million) for grants to projects for expanding the number of farmers' markets accepting food stamp electronic benefit transfer (EBT) cards.

Geographic Preference and Buy American Rules

- As in the House bill, generally overrode current rules that limit the extent to which schools and the DOD Fresh program can specify a geographic preference (e.g., for locally produced food items) when procuring food for meals served by child nutrition providers.
- Similar to the House bill, encouraged implementation of existing Buy American requirements for child nutrition programs.

Puerto Rico

- As in the House bill, directed a comprehensive study of extending the regular Food Stamp program to Puerto Rico as a state (in lieu of its nutrition assistance block grant). Also provided mandatory funding of $1 million for the study.
- Similar to the House bill, revamped and replaced current provisions of law governing Emerson-Leland hunger fellowships. Authorized appropriations of such sums as are necessary.

Health and Nutrition Promotion Projects

- Required the establishment of pilot projects to develop, test, and evaluate methods of using the Food Stamp program to improve the dietary and health status of participating households and to reduce overweight, obesity, and associated diet-related diseases. Among other initiatives, projects could include those increasing program benefits; expanding access to farmers' markets; providing incentives to vendors to increase the availability of healthy foods; adding vendor requirements with respect to carrying healthy foods; supporting nutrition/health education programs; and providing recipients with point-of-purchase financial incentives to encourage purchase of fruits, vegetables, and other healthy foods. Mandatory funding of $50 million was provided for these projects, the largest portion of which was set aside for point-of-purchase incentive pilots.

Hunger-Free Communities: Studies and Grants[48]

- Required a periodically updated study of major matters relating to the problem of hunger in the United States, assessing data and hunger-reduction measures that have been and could be carried out, as well as making recommendations for policies to reduce hunger.
- Authorized matching grants (1) to food program service providers and nonprofit organizations to assess community hunger problems and meet goals for achieving "hunger-free communities" and (2) to emergency feeding organizations for infrastructure development.
- Authorized appropriations of $50 million a year for these studies and grants.

Bill Emerson and Mickey Leland Hunger Fellows

- Similar to the House bill, revamped and replaced current provisions of law governing Emerson-Leland hunger fellowships. Authorized appropriations of such sums as are necessary.

Enrolling Children for Free School Meals

- Required assessment of (and annual reports on) the effectiveness of each state in enrolling children in food stamp households for free school meals using "direct certification" procedures.

Periodic Surveys

- Required periodic surveys of foods purchased by schools in the School Lunch program and provided mandatory funding of $3 million for each survey.

Nutrition Monitoring

- As in the House bill, required continuation of national nutrition monitoring activities.

Team Nutrition Network

- Provided mandatory funding of $3 million a year (through FY2012) for Team Nutrition (education) Network activities authorized under the Child Nutrition Act.

Agriculture Policy and Public Health

- Required the Government Accountability Office (GAO) to assess whether the agricultural policies of the U.S. have an impact on health, nutrition, overweight, obesity, and diet-related disease.

Whole Grain Pilot Project

- Established a pilot project to provide whole grain products in selected elementary and secondary schools. Provided funding of $4 million a year drawn from money available for Senior Farmers' Market Nutrition programs and Community Food projects.

Report on Federal Hunger Programs

- Required the GAO to submit a report that surveys all federal programs seeking to alleviate hunger or food insecurity or to improve nutritional intake.

Food Employment Empowerment and Development Program[49]

- Authorized a "food employment empowerment and development program" under which grants would be made to encourage the effective use of community resources to combat hunger and the causes of hunger through food recovery and job training initiatives.

Infrastructure and Transportation Grants

- Authorized competitive grants, totaling $10 million a year through FY20 12, to expand the capacity and infrastructure of food banks in rural areas and improve their ability to handle "time-sensitive" (perishable) foods.

The Enacted 2008 Farm Bill

After two vetoes (overridden by Congress), the farm bill, entitled the Food, Conservation, and Energy Act of 2008, became law, as P.L. 110-246, on June 18, 2008.[50] The new Act's nutrition title (Title IV) covers (extends or amends) the Food Stamp program, The Emergency Food Assistance Program (TEFAP), the fresh fruit and vegetable program in schools, the Senior Farmers' Market program, programs in lieu of food stamps in Puerto Rico and American Samoa and on Indian reservations, the Commodity Supplemental Food Program, rules governing procurement of food for school meal programs, congressional hunger fellowships, and various special nutrition projects. It includes the extensions of authority for and changes in domestic nutrition assistance laws noted below.[51]

While, as with the House and Senate bills, many provisions do not have a direct cost effect, several important revisions do. The Congressional Budget Office (the CBO) estimate of the total new spending expected from Title IV initiatives varies according to which "baseline" (i.e., costs with no changes in law) assumptions are used and the time period over which costs are projected. Spending figures also differ depending on whether offsetting reductions are taken into account.

Under pre-2008 law, the programs covered by Title IV were anticipated to cost (in outlays) approximately $186 billion over FY2008-FY2012 (the 5-year "life" of the 2008 farm bill) and almost $400 billion over the 10-year span from FY2008 to FY2017, using the CBO March 2007 baseline. Projecting from the CBO March 2008 baseline, Title IV programs were expected to cost about $206 billion over FY2008- FY2012 and just over $430 billion over FY2008-FY2017. Taken as a percentage increase over these baseline amounts, Title IV provisions are expected to add between 1% and 2% in new spending (outlays) over 5 years and just over 2% over 10 years (see below).

Using the March 2007 CBO baseline — this baseline was employed by Congress in making decisions as to the provisions to be included in Title IV, and estimates using it are those most often cited in describing the effects of the farm bill — the CBO estimates project total net Title IV costs (outlays) at $2.897 billion over FY2008-FY2012 and $9.218 billion over FY2008-FY2017. On the other hand, if the March 2008 baseline is used, total net Title IV costs increase to $3.11 billion over FY2008-FY2012 and $9.66 billion over FY2008-FY2017. These net cost estimates (under *both* baseline assumptions) do *not* include new spending for the Fresh Fruit and Vegetable program (see below) that are effectively offset with money from permanent "Section 32"[52] appropriations provided through an amendment (Section 14222) in

Title XIV of the new law — that is, $274 million (FY2008-FY2012) and $1.02 billion (FY2008-FY2017).

Six provisions of the enacted law account for virtually all of the cost of the provisions of Title IV: (1) increasing food stamp benefits by raising the "standard deduction" disregard of income, (2) boosting food stamp benefits by eliminating limits on income disregards tied to dependent care expenses, (3) raising minimum food stamp benefits, (4) increasing food stamp dollar limits on allowable liquid assets and disregarding retirement savings/plans and education savings as countable assets when judging food stamp eligibility, (5) increasing mandatory spending on TEFAP commodities, and (6) expanding support for the fresh fruit and vegetable program in schools. The large majority of new spending generated by the changes incorporated in Title IV is tied to changes in food stamp law.

The nutrition title of the enacted farm bill responds to the overwhelming majority of proposals for change put forward in bills pending before Congress and supported by the advocacy community (all of which call for various program expansions and new initiatives). It includes no program cutbacks and very few of the Administration's recommendations. Only three significant pieces of the Administration's nutrition title package are accepted: the disregard of retirement plans/savings and education savings when judging food stamp eligibility, lifting limits on dependent-care cost disregards, and changing rules governing the treatment of retailers violating food stamp rules. However, while the nutrition title includes most of the provisions for added benefits, loosened eligibility standards, and new or expanded nutrition program initiatives, it does not necessarily adopt the most expansive approaches to these changes — primarily because of cost concerns.

Food Stamps

General Provisions

- Renames the Food Stamp Program and the Food Stamp Act as the Supplemental Nutrition Assistance Program (SNAP) and the Food and Nutrition Act.
- Makes coupons issued under the Food Stamp program — prior to the changeover to electronic benefit transfer (EBT) cards as of method of issuing benefits — no longer redeemable.

Benefit Levels and Eligibility

- Increases benefits (and, to a limited degree, liberalizes income eligibility standards) for most households by raising and then indexing the minimum amount of household monthly income that is disregarded (the "standard deduction") by calculating benefits (and, to a limited degree, income eligibility). The monthly minimum standard deduction is initially increased to $144 (for FY2009), and then annually increased for inflation in later years. This change accounts for just over half the cost of the provisions in the nutrition title.
- Increases benefits (and, to a limited degree, liberalizes income eligibility standards) for some households with dependent or child care expenses by removing dollar limits on the degree to which these expenses are taken into account.
- Increases minimum benefits by calculating them as 8% of the (indexed) maximum monthly benefit for a one-person household.

- Places into permanent law a rule that disregards combat-related pay for families with military members when calculating benefits and eligibility.
- Bars food stamp eligibility to those disqualified from the FDPIR.
- Allows states to provide "transitional" food stamp benefits to households with children that cease to receive cash assistance under a state-funded public assistance program.
- Disqualifies persons found to have intentionally (1) obtained cash by misusing program benefits to obtain money for the return of deposits on containers or (2) sold food purchased with program benefits.

Asset Eligibility Standards

- Increases the degree to which liquid assets are disregarded when judging eligibility by indexing the dollar limits on assets for inflation.
- Adds to the list of assets that are to be disregarded all tax-recognized retirement plans/savings and education savings.

Program Administration

- Requires standards for identifying major changes in state agency administrative operations and mandates that, if a state implements a major change in operations, it must notify the Agriculture Department and collect any information needed to identify and correct any adverse effects on program integrity or access.
- Requires that computerized systems for state agency operations must be tested adequately before and after implementation and be operated under a plan for continuous updating and testing.
- Permits the Agriculture Department to make a determination that a state agency has over-issued benefits to a substantial number of households because of a "major systemic error" by the state. If this determination is made, the Department may (1) prohibit the state agency from collecting any resulting over-issuances from recipients and (2) collect the cost of over-issuances from the state.
- Expands the application of "simplified reporting" rules by allowing states to extend periodic reporting of changes in household circumstances (as opposed to reporting all changes when they occur) to households with elderly or disabled members (and certain others).
- Allows households to accrue unused benefits under the electronic benefit transfer system.
- Requires consistent federally established procedures for identifying felons fleeing from active pursuit for prosecution or custody.
- Places into law specific rules governing the use of "telephonic signatures" for food stamp applications.
- Limits "split issuance" of benefits by requiring that no staggered issuance procedure may provide for more than 1 issuance during a month, expect in the case of a benefit correction.
- Allows "job retention services" to be provided to those who have obtained employment as part of an employment/training program and allows volunteers for employment and training to participate for more than the normal maximum of 20 hours a week.

- Expands privacy protections for applicants and recipients to control the release of information obtained from them to third parties.
- Limits the time that unspent federal funding for expenses of employment and training programs can remain available.

Retailers

- Revises rules with regard to penalties on retailers for violations of food stamp law or regulations: (1) allows fines of up to $100,000 per violation, (2) permits imposition of both a disqualification and a money penalty, and (3) removes minimum disqualification periods.
- Bars charging retailers "interchange fees" in connection with implementation of electronic benefit transfer systems.

Other Provisions and Programs

Reauthorization

- Generally extends expiring authorities in the (renamed) Food Stamp Act and other laws governing programs covered in the nutrition title (including authorizations of appropriations and spending directives) through FY20 12. Amendments are made part of permanent law.

The Emergency Food Assistance Program (TEFAP)

- Increases mandatory funding for TEFAP commodities. For FY2008, an immediate infusion of $50 million is directed. For FY2009, $250 million in TEFAP commodities is mandated, up from $140 million under prior law. For FY20 10 through FY20 12, the $250 million provided for FY2009 is to be adjusted for food-price inflation.
- Increases the annual authorization of appropriations for TEFAP administrative and distribution costs to $100 million.
- Authorizes appropriations ($15 million a year) for TEFAP "infrastructure grants."

Fruits and Vegetables

- Replaces the existing program supporting the offering of fresh fruits and vegetables in schools, beginning with the 2008-2009 school year. The new initiative will provide funding for the program to operate in elementary schools selected by states. New mandatory funding of $40 million (for FY2008) is provided, followed by $65 million for the 2009-20 10 school year, $101 million for the 20 10- 2011 school year, and $150 million for the 2011-2012 school year. Available money for each succeeding school year is indexed for inflation. Funding is made available through provisions in Title XIV of the enacted law. Money is allocated to states under a formula distributing about half the money equally among states and apportioning the remainder on the basis of state population. Priority is to be given to schools that have high proportions of low-income students, and states are responsible for selecting schools and must limit annual per-student grants to $50-$75. Provides funding for an evaluation of this effort and allows limited set-asides for federal and state administrative costs.

- Provides that, in addition to the minimum ($200 million-a-year) acquisition of fruits, vegetables, and nuts for use in domestic food assistance programs required under the 2002 farm bill, the Agriculture Department will purchase additional fruits, vegetables, and nuts for use in these programs. Added acquisitions are required to be $190 million (FY2008), $193 million (FY2009), $199 million (FY20 10), $203 million (FY20 1 1), and $206 million (FY20 12 and each year thereafter). Retains a requirement for a $50-million-a-year purchase of fresh fruits and vegetables for schools (currently carried out through Defense Department procurement facilities under the "DoD Fresh" program).

Commodity Supplemental Food Program (CSFP)

- Bars the Agriculture Department from requiring that CSFP projects prioritize assistance among the elderly or women, infants, and children, but does not change eligibility rules.

Food Distribution Program on Indian Reservations (FDPIR)

- Authorizes funding ($5 million a year) for a fund to purchase "traditional and locally grown foods" for the FDPIR, mandates that at least half of these foods are to be from Native American farmers, ranchers, and producers, and authorizes funding for bison meat purchases for the FDPIR.
- Requires a report reviewing the procedures for determining the contents of FDPIR food packages and a survey of participants as to their preference among traditional foods.

Senior Farmers' Market Nutrition Program (SFMNP)

- Increases total mandatory funding for the SFMNP to $20.6 million a year (from $15 million annually).
- Adds honey to the items that may be purchased with SFMNP vouchers.
- Bars consideration of SFMNP benefits as income/resources in for tax purposes and in other public aid programs and prohibits the collection of sales taxes on SFMNP purchases.

Farmers' Markets and EBT Cards

- Provides mandatory funding ($5 million) for grants to projects for expanding the number of farmers' markets that accept electronic benefit transfer (EBT) cards. This provision is included in Title X of the enacted law.

Community Food Projects

- Requires a grant to a nonprofit organization to establish and support a "healthy urban food enterprise development center" to carry out activities that increase access to healthy affordable foods (including locally produced food) in "underserved communities." Mandatory funding of $1 million a year is made available.
- Authorizes a new pilot program to provide grants to high-poverty schools for initiatives in hands-on gardening.

Geographic Preference (Purchase of Locally Produced Foods)

- Requires the Agriculture Department to allow schools and other institutions receiving funds under the National School Lunch and Child Nutrition Acts (and the Defense Department acting as a fresh fruit and vegetable buying agent) to use geographic preference for the procurement of "unprocessed agricultural products, both locally grown and locally raised."

Puerto Rico

- Directs a comprehensive study of extending the regular Food Stamp program (renamed the Supplemental Nutrition Assistance program) to Puerto Rico as a state (in lieu of its nutrition assistance block grant). Provides $1 million to carry out the study.

Health and Nutrition Promotion Projects

- Authorizes pilot projects that develop and test methods of using the (renamed) Food Stamp program to improve the dietary and health status of participants and eligible persons and reduce overweight, obesity, and diet-related diseases. Provides mandatory funding ($20 million) for "point-of-purchase incentive" projects that carry out this initiative.

Hunger-Free Communities Grants

- Authorizes matching grants (1) to food program service providers and nonprofits for efforts to assess community hunger problems and to achieve "hunger-free communities" and (2) to emergency feeding organizations for infrastructure development.

Foods Purchased by Schools

- Requires a survey of foods purchased by schools in child nutrition programs and provides mandatory funding for the survey ($3 million).

Whole Grain Pilot Project

- Requires the Agriculture Department to purchase whole grains and whole grain products for use in school meal programs. Includes a directive for an evaluation of this project and provides $4 million to carry out the project (funding is provided in Title XIV of the enacted law).

Enrolling Children for Free School Meals

- Requires periodic assessments of states' effectiveness in enrolling children in food stamp households for free school meals using "direct certification" procedures.

Bill Emerson and Mickey Leland Congressional Hunger Fellowships

- Revises provisions authorizing a Congressional Hunger Fellowship program and authorizes appropriations at "such sums as are necessary."

References

[1] For a look at the farm bill as a whole, see CRS Report RL3 3934, *The 2008 Farm Bill: A Summary of Major Provisions and Legislative Action*, coordinated by Renee Johnson.

[2] Normally, the only child-nutrition or WIC-related provisions that might appear in a farm bill are those relating to commodity assistance to schools or initiatives like fresh fruit and vegetable projects, discussed later in this report. However, past farm bills have, in some cases, included relatively minor revisions affecting child nutrition and WIC program operations. Child nutrition and WIC programs were last subject to a comprehensive review and reauthorization in the 2004 Child Nutrition and WIC Reauthorization Act (P.L. 108- 265). Unlike in the Senate, where they (along with most other food assistance programs) are under the jurisdiction of the Senate Committee on Agriculture, Nutrition, and Forestry, child nutrition and WIC programs are in the jurisdiction of the Education and Labor Committee in the House.

[3] Major exceptions are funding levels for the Commodity Supplemental Food Program (the CSFP) and the Food Distribution Program on Indian Reservations (the FDPIR) — both set in the annual appropriations process. In addition, Agriculture Department appropriations bills sometimes include legislative changes; for those being considered in the FY2008 appropriations process, see CRS Report RL34 132, *Agriculture and Related Agencies: FY2008 Appropriations*, coordinated by Jim Monke.

[4] For domestic food assistance in the USDA budget, see CRS Report RL34 132, *Agriculture and Related Agencies: FY2008 Appropriations*, coordinated by Jim Monke.

[5] Nutrition programs for the elderly (authorized under the Older Americans Act and administered through the Department of Health and Human Services) are the only domestic nutrition assistance programs outside the USDA. They are typically funded at about $700 million a year in the appropriations measure for the Department of Health and Human Services.[1] For a look at the farm bill as a whole, see CRS Report RL3 3934, *The 2008 Farm Bill: A Summary of Major Provisions and Legislative Action*, coordinated by Renee Johnson.

[6] For a detailed discussion of nutrition assistance program changes made and considered in the 2002 farm bill, see CRS Report RL3 3690, *Food Stamps and Nutrition Programs in the 2002 Farm Bill*, by Joe Richardson.

[7] Authorized under the Food Stamp Act; 7 U.S.C. 2011 et seq.

[8] A dollar in food stamp benefits is estimated to result in new food spending of 17-47 cents, depending on household income and type, versus 5-10 cents in the case of a dollar of cash. Although food stamp aid itself must be spent on food, a dollar in food stamps does not lead to a full dollar of additional food spending because cash previously spent on food is freed up and can be used for nonfood expenses that, for the recipient, may be more pressing.

[9] This second category was denominated as "food insecure with hunger" in reports for earlier years. Households classified as "food insecure" were grouped into two

categories. Those classified as having "low food security" (7.1%) reported multiple indications of food access problems, but typically reported few, if any, indications of reduced food intake. Those classified as having "very low food security" (3.9%) reported multiple indications of reduced food intake and disrupted eating patterns due to inadequate resources for food.

[10] Alaska and Hawaii, along with the Virgin Islands and Guam to a lesser extent, are special exceptions to this general rule.

[11] To put these participation figures into perspective, it should be noted that the all-time high in food stamp participation was reached shortly before enactment of the 1996 welfare reform law — 27.5 million persons a month in FY1994. The all-time low for the modern program was in FY2000 — 17.2 million persons a month.

[12] Information on error rates and fraud ("trafficking" in food stamp benefits) can be found in two recent Government Accountability Office (GAO) reports: *Food Stamp Program: States Have Made Progress Reducing Payment Errors, and Further Challenges Remain* (GAO-05-245; May 2005) and *Food Stamp Trafficking: FNS Could Enhance Program Integrity by Better Targeting Stores Likely to Traffic and Increasing Penalties* (GAO-07-53; October 2006).

[13] Information on state options can be found in a 2004 GAO report — Food Stamp Program: Farm Bill Options Ease Administrative Burdens, but Opportunities Exist to Streamline Participant Reporting Rules among Programs (GAO-04-916; September 2004); available at [http://www.gao.gov/new.items/d049 16.pdf]. Coverage of the current status of state options is on the USDA website at [http://www.fns.usda.gov/fsp/rules/Memo/Support/State_ Options/7-State_Options.pdf]. And information about states' use of their options as to how to count the value of vehicles when determining food stamp eligibility can be found in a report by the Center on Budget and Policy Priorities — State Vehicle Asset Policies in the Food Stamp Program (revised November 6, 2006) — available through the Center's website: [http://www.cbpp.org].

[14] A fuller discussion can be found in a report — *Administration Proposal Would Cut Over 300,000 People Off Food Stamps* — from the Center on Budget and Policy Priorities, available at the Center's website: [http://www.cbpp.org].

[15] A fuller discussion can be found in a report — *Families' Food Stamp Benefits Purchase Less Food Each Year* — from the Center on Budget and Policy Priorities, available at the Center's website: [http://www.cbpp.org].

[16] Florida's project is effectively fully implemented; Indiana is in the process of implementing its initiative; Texas has, for the time-being, put a stop to its project.

[17] A more extensive discussion of the Administration's proposals is available in CRS Report RL339 16, *The USDA 2007 Farm Bill Proposal: Possible Questions*, coordinated by Jasper Womach.

[18] At present, states are only penalized for high rates of error in overpaying or underpaying benefits.

[19] It would also "de-obligate" the few food stamp coupons still in circulation, making them no longer usable (redeemable).

[20] Nutrition education activities are already eligible for 50% federal funding as a state administrative expense.

[21] Authorized under Section 19 of the Food Stamp Act; 7 U.S.C. 2028.
[22] Authorized under Section 4(b) of the Food Stamp Act; 7 U.S.C. 20 13(b).
[23] No extension was necessary for the Northern Marianas grant because it operates under a separate permanent authorization.
[24] Authorized under (1) Section 27 of the Food Stamp Act (7 U.S.C. 2036) and (2) the Emergency Food Assistance Act (7 U.S.C. 7501-75 16).
[25] Typically $ 10-$20 million a year.
[26] Authorized under Sections 4 and 5 of the Agriculture and Consumer Protection Act of 1973; 7 U.S.C. 612c note.
[27] For FY2008, the Agriculture Department appropriations law actually includes a significant increase in CSFP appropriations.
[28] In Section 4402 of the 2002 farm bill.
[29] A more extensive discussion of the Administration's proposals for fruit and vegetable purchase policies is available in CRS Report RL33916, *The USDA 2007 Farm Bill Proposal: Possible Questions*, coordinated by Jasper Womach.
[30] These rules are intended to encourage expansion of the summer program by freeing program sponsors from a requirement that they provide detailed documentation of their expenses.
[31] This bill also includes related provisions that are outside the typical purview of child nutrition laws. They authorize a pilot program of grants to schools to increase the length of school days for physical activity and other initiatives.
[32] A similar measure was approved by the Senate on December 8, 2006.
[33] For information on the FY2008 appropriation , see CRS Report RL34 132, *Agriculture and Related Ag[3]encies: FY2008 Appropriations*, coordinated by Jim Monke.
[34] See S. 790/H.R. 1740.
[35] For a longer discussion of extensions of expiring authorities and the farm bill, see CRS Report RL33934, *The 2008 Farm Bill: A Summary of Major Provisions and Legislative Action,* coordinated by Renee Johnson.
[36] This represents a 2.2% increase over the most current (March 2007) Congressional Budget Office "baseline" estimate of spending under current law for programs under the nutrition title over the next five years ($192.2 billion).
[37] *Note:* Income disregard provisions primarily affect benefit calculations. However, they can affect a household's income eligibility. Most households are subject to both a "gross" income test — their total income, *before* disregards (deductions), must be below 130% of the federal poverty income guidelines — and a "net" income test — their income, *after* disregards (deductions), must be below the poverty guidelines themselves. In the overwhelming majority of situations, meeting the gross income test is the more important requirement. But boosting or establishing an income disregard also decreases a household's net income and can make their income eligibility more likely. Elderly or disabled households are subject only to a net income test.
[38] Current limits are $200 a month for children under age 2 and $175 a month for all other dependents. This proposal also was put forward by the Administration, among others.

[39] This proposal also was put forward by the Administration, among others, and is included in the FY2008 Agriculture Department appropriations measure.

[40] Asset limits are now set at $2,000, or $3,000 for households with an elderly or disabled member.

[41] This proposal was put forward by the Administration, among others.

[42] See the discussion of the Senate bill for more detail.

[43] Current provisions have not been implemented. Instead, the hunger fellowship program continues to receive annual appropriations ($2.5 million in FY2006 and proposed for FY2008) from Congress, without any specific legislative guidance as to their use.

[44] This represents a 2.8% increase over the Congressional Budget Office "baseline" estimate of spending under current law for programs under the nutrition title over the next five years ($192.2 billion).

[45] *Note:* Income disregard provisions primarily affect benefit calculations. However, they also can affect a household's income eligibility to some extent. See footnote 38 for a fuller discussion.

[46] Current limits are $200 a month for children under age 2 and $175 a month for all other dependents. This proposal was put forward by the Administration, among others.

[47] This proposal also was put forward by the Administration, among others. It is included in the FY2008 Agriculture Department appropriations measure.

[48] Also see S. 1172, entitled the Hunger-Free Communities Act.

[49] See S. 1575.

[50] See CRS Report RL33934, *The 2008 Farm Bill: A Summary of Major Provisions and Legislative Action*, coordinated by Renee Johnson, for details on House and Senate action on the conference agreement (H.Rept. 110-627), the Presidential vetoes, and various extensions of expiring authorities pending the Farm Bill's enactment.

[51] For additional details on the enacted farm bill's Title IV, see the website of the Center on Budget and Policy Priorities at [http://www.cbpp.org].

[52] For information on Section 32, see CRS Report RL34081, *Farm and Food Support under* USDA's Section 32 Program, by Geoffrey Becker.

In: Hunger in America: Issues and Assistance
Editor: Gaston T. LaBue, pp. 67-79
ISBN: 978-1-60692-803-5

Chapter 3

CHARITABLE CONTRIBUTIONS OF FOOD INVENTORY: PROPOSALS FOR CHANGE*

Pamela J. Jackson

ABSTRACT

Tax law provides an enhanced deduction for certain charitable contributions of food inventory. The value of the existing deduction is the corporation's basis in the donated product plus one half of the amount of appreciation, as long as that amount is less than twice the basis in the product. This deduction has generally been limited to contributions made by a certain type of corporation, C corporations.

Although the temporary expansion of the enhanced deduction may have the effect of reducing equity differences between C corporations and other business concerns, it may not entirely eliminate them. If the intent is to resolve the equity issues, transforming the deduction to a credit might be more effective. Unlike deductions, whose value is based on the tax rate of the taxpayer, tax credits provide dollar-for-dollar value and do not fluctuate with the taxpayer's marginal tax bracket.

This report will be updated to reflect major legislative developments.

This report discusses the temporary change in the tax law governing charitable donations of food. Recent legislation expanded the existing tax incentive for firms that are C corporations to all businesses that donate food to charity.

In response to the devastation from Hurricane Katrina, the Katrina Emergency Tax Relief Act of 2005 (KETRA, P.L. 109-73) was enacted. That legislation included a temporary expansion of the tax deduction for charitable contributions of food inventory. The law allowed all donors of wholesome food inventory to benefit from the enhanced deduction for donations made between August 28, 2005, and January 1, 2006. The Pension Protection Act of 2006 (P.L. 109-280) extended the temporary expansion through January 1, 2008.

* Excerpted from CRS Report RL31097, dated August 22, 2008.

In the 110th Congress, the Good Samaritan Hunger Relief Tax Incentive Extension Act of 2007 (S. 689) proposes to permanently extend and expand the charitable deduction for contributions of food inventory. H.R. 3976 proposes making the provision permanent.

H.R. 3996, the Temporary Tax Relief Act of 2007, and H.R. 6049, the Renewable Energy and Job Creation Act of 2008, which were passed by the House, both include a provision to retroactively extend the temporary expansion of eligible donors through December 31, 2008, as do H.R. 3970, the Tax Reduction and Reform Act of 2007; S. 3335, the Jobs, Energy, Families, and Disaster Relief Act of 2008; and S. 3125, the Energy Independence and Tax Relief Act of 2008.

Proposals to retroactively extend the temporary expansion of eligible donors through December 31, 2009, have been made in S. 2886, the Alternative Minimum Tax and Extenders Tax Relief Act of 2008; S. 3098, also titled the Alternative Minimum Tax and Extenders Tax Relief Act of 2008; and S. 3322 and its companion H.R. 6587, the Midwestern Disaster Tax Relief Act of 2008. H.R. 3628, the Promoting Charitable Actions Act of 2007, proposes extension through 2011.

Additionally, S. 1132 proposes to qualify Indian tribes as eligible recipients of tax deductible contributions of food inventory.

S. 2420, the Federal Food Donation Act of 2008, which became law in June 2008 (P.L. 110-247), revised the Federal Acquisition Regulation to require certain contracts to private entities to include a clause that encourages the donation of food. Specifically, the law requires that all contracts above $25,000 for the provision, services, or sale of food in the United States, or for the lease or rental of Federal property to a private entity for events at which food is provided in the United States, shall include a clause that encourages the donation of excess, apparently wholesome food to nonprofit organizations that provide assistance to food-insecure people.[1] The legislation does not address the tax treatment of those donations.

TAX LAW

A discussion of the tax treatment for contributions made by all types of businesses is provided. Generally, these contributions may be made only to certain types of nonprofit organizations, may be deductible for income tax purposes only up to specified limits, and may be in the form of either cash or property. The charitable contribution deduction is allowed only for the taxable year in which the contribution is made; any unpaid subscriptions or pledges are not deductible until actually fulfilled.

Some of the more typical organizations to which contributions are deductible include churches, universities, schools, and hospitals, as well as many other public assistance charities (such as food pantries, soup kitchens, homeless shelters, etc). If a contribution is made to an individual, such as a homeless family living on the street, that contribution is not deductible even though actuated by charitable motives.

In order to qualify as an organization to which contributions are deductible, the recipient must be organized or incorporated in the United States or in one of its possessions and certified as a charitable organization by the Internal Revenue Service.[2] Contributions to foreign charitable organizations are not deductible. A donation, however, to an otherwise qualified organization is deductible even though some portion of the funds of such organization are used in foreign countries for charity.

Limitation on the Amount Deductible

The deduction for contributions (either in cash or in property) made by corporations is limited to 10% of taxable income (computed with adjustments). The 10% cap was raised from 5% by the passage of the *Economic Recovery Tax Act of 1981*. The legislative history of the 1981 Act indicates that Congress was hopeful that corporate charitable contributions would be stimulated by the increase in the cap.

Carryforward

Although the deductible portion of any contribution by corporations may not exceed 10% of taxable income in any given year, if contributions exceed this limitation, the excess may be carried forward to future tax years. Corporations may carry over excess charitable contributions and compute tax as though the excess gifts were actually made in such subsequent years. Thus, when charitable contributions in one year exceed the limitation, a corporation might ultimately secure the full benefit (taxwise) of the contribution even though denied part of it in the year in which the contribution was initially made. The law allows that excess charitable contributions may be carried forward for a five-year period. This carryforward provision applies to both gifts of cash or property.

Contributions of Property — Including Food Products

In general, if a charitable contribution is made in the form of property, the basis for the charitable deduction is dependent on the type of taxpayer (i.e., individual or form of business entity), to whom the property is donated, and for what purpose the donated property is to be used.

Corporate gifts of property that would generate capital gains if sold (e.g., stocks and bonds) are deductible by corporations at market value. However, gifts of depreciable property are deductible at the corporation's basis rather than fair market value. Thus, under current tax law, the deduction is reduced by previously taken depreciation. In the case of fully depreciated machinery and equipment, the allowable charitable contribution deduction would be zero.

Under current tax law, C corporations[3] are provided more favorable tax treatment of contributions of certain types of inventory and other ordinary-income property to specified charitable organizations. This provision is temporarily available to S corporations[4], partnerships, and sole proprietorships. Through 2007, all donors are allowed to deduct their cost plus one-half the difference between their cost and the market value of the donated goods. However, in no case may the deduction's value exceed twice the cost basis. This special tax inducement is provided for capital assets defined in Internal Revenue Code § 1221(1) or (2).[5] Thus, this provision allows very large corporations a bigger deduction for charitable contributions of qualified tangible personal property.

For a donor to receive this enhanced deduction, the gift must be made to a "qualified" tax exempt organization.[6] Further, the property must be "used by the donee solely for the care of the ill, the needy, or infants."[7] The donee is not permitted to exchange what has been transferred for money, other property, or services.[8] The donee must furnish the donor with a statement that it does not intend to transfer the donation and that it will be used for the care of the ill, the needy, or infants.[9] If the property is subject to regulation by the Federal Food, Drug, and Cosmetic Act it must satisfy the requirements on the date of transfer and for 180 days prior thereto.[10]

The enhanced deduction for food is available only for food that qualifies as "apparently wholesome food." "Apparently wholesome food" is defined under the Katrina Emergency Tax Relief Act of 2005 (KETRA) as food intended for human consumption that meets all quality and labeling standards imposed by federal, state, and local laws and regulations even though the food may not be readily marketable due to appearance, age, freshness, grade, size, surplus, or other conditions.

Summary of Restrictions

In summary, current law provides that the charitable deduction for contributions of inventory and other property is as follows:

- The gift must be made to a U.S. charitable organization;
- There is a 10% limitation on the total amount a corporation can deduct as charitable contributions;
- Contributions made in excess of this limitation may be carried forward for the next five years;
- Special rules are available for gifts made by C corporations of tangible personal property (inventory) when donated to qualified charitable organizations for the care of the ill, the needy, or infants.
- It must be established that the fair market value of the product exceeds basis in order to use the enhanced deduction.

Past Legislative Proposals

As noted earlier in this report, current law provides an enhanced deduction for donations made by C Corporations of property, which includes food products, for the care of the ill, the needy, or infants. This enhanced deduction available for food products is used primarily by businesses for unsaleable products. The most frequent reasons for products not being sold at market are errors in labeling, merchandise that has been crushed or dented, or products that may be too close to the expiration date recommended for sale.

There have been four parts to legislation proposing to change the tax law for donated food products, two of which were addressed in the 109th Congress. Typically, the proposals would extend the enhanced deduction for food inventory to all taxpayers engaged in a trade or business. Secondly, the enhanced deduction would be available only for "apparently wholesome food" which is newly defined under some of the legislative proposals. Third, the determination of basis of the qualified contributions would be set as a percentage of the food's fair market value. Finally, some proposals have set the fair market value of donated foods to be the same price as similar food items sold by the taxpayer at the time of the contribution, or, in the recent past.

Apparently Wholesome Food

Typically, legislative proposals have defined "apparently wholesome food" to include food that "may not be readily marketable due to appearance, age, freshness, grade, size, surplus, or other conditions." The new law provides a slightly more rigorous definition. The inclusion of the definition and the discussion of how fair market value is to be determined is designed to lessen valuation problems for taxpayers caused by a lack of clarity in the regulations.

A court case in the 9th Circuit was also at odds with the regulations regarding donation valuation as issued by the Internal Revenue Service and the findings in that case clarified the issue. The court case held that the value of surplus bread inventory donated to a qualified charity was determined to be the same as the full retail price of the bread.[11] The Internal Revenue Service (IRS) contended that the retail value of the bread was half the normal sales price since the industry practice of major bakers is to discount four-day-old bread, but if the court had ruled the value of the bread was half the retail selling price, the donor would have received no tax benefit and, thus, no encouragement to make such charitable donations.[12] The court's findings contradicted regulations issued by IRS.

The new definition of "apparently wholesome food" parallels the definition included in the Bill Emerson Good Samaritan Food Donation Act (42 U.S.C. 179 1(b)(2)). That act defines the term "apparently wholesome food" as food that meets all quality and labeling standards imposed by federal, state, and local laws and regulations even though the food may not be readily marketable due to appearance, age, freshness, grade, size, surplus, or other conditions. This definition was also used in the temporary law enacted by the Katrina Emergency Relief Act (P.L. 109-7 3).

ABBREVIATED HISTORY

Prior to the passage of the *Tax Reform Act of 1969*, the general rule was that taxpayers who contributed appreciated property to charities were allowed a charitable contribution for the fair market value of the property. Moreover, no tax was imposed or collected on the appreciation. As an example, a farmer making a charitable contribution of a portion of his crop not only received a tax deduction of the fair market value of the donated crops, but also escaped the tax on the difference between his crop production costs and fair market value. Because the tax savings from the charitable deduction (in the case of ordinary income property) was measured by the taxpayer's marginal tax rate, it was possible for taxpayers to make contributions which permitted a greater after-tax benefit than would have been received if the crop had been sold and the farmer allowed to keep the proceeds after paying tax on the gain. It should be remembered that tax rates at that time were much higher than today's rates. Since this provision was seen as unfair when compared with those making charitable cash gifts, the Tax Reform Act of 1969 changed the law so that the appreciated value was to result in a reduction of the contribution deduction to the extent of the appreciation.

It was with passage of the *Tax Reform Act of 1976* (P.L. 94-455) that corporations were provided more favorable tax treatment of contributions of inventory (such as food) to certain charitable organizations. The 1976 Act provided that such gifts by corporations were to be based on the taxpayer's basis in the property and one-half of the unrealized appreciation as long as the deduction did not exceed twice the property's basis.[13] In a summary of the act, it was stated that the enactment of the Tax Reform Act of 1969 had resulted in reduced contributions of certain types of property to charitable institutions. In particular, those charitable organizations that provide food, clothing, medical equipment, and supplies, etc. to the needy and disaster victims had found that contributions of such items to those organizations were reduced.[14] It was stated in the general explanation of the law that Congress believed that it was desirable to provide a greater tax incentive than in prior law for contributions of certain types of ordinary income property which the donee charity uses in the performance of its exempt purposes. However, Congress believed that the deduction allowed should not be such that the donor could be in a better after-tax situation by donating the property than by selling it.[15]

STATISTICAL TRENDS

In 2006, total charitable giving was estimated to have reached $295 billion. Corporations and their foundations contributed $12.7 billion in cash and in-kind donations. Two predictors of corporate giving, corporate pretax profits and the gross domestic product both rose in 2006. Individual giving represented 75.6% of total giving and corporate gifts were 4.3% of the total (with foundations and bequests representing the remainder). However, these numbers mask the importance of corporate charitable gifts because religious organizations receive little funding from either corporate donors or their foundations since individuals are the primary support of religious institutions. The American Association of Fund-Raising Counsel (AAFRC) Trust for Philanthropy, Inc. found that for 2006, contributions to religion represented 32.8% of all charitable gifts.[16] It is important to remember that companies support non-profits through cause-related marketing, public relations, sponsorships, contracts, and other joint promotional activities as well as through advertising expenditures. These types of expenditures are not shown as charitable gifts. In an earlier edition of *Giving USA*, the AAFRC Trust for Philanthropy, Inc. made the following four points:

- Corporate giving has ranged from a low point of 0.7% to a high of 2.3% of pretax income over 30 years, with historical variation largely due to changes in tax law.
- Profits grow fastest in the service industries, like banking and telecommunications. Non-manufacturing companies cannot take advantage of tax-deductible gifts of inventory that make up much of the manufacturing sector's charitable activity, even though non- manufacturers make up a large component of profit growth.
- There is a trend toward strategic corporate support, which is not counted as a charitable gift by the company, the IRS, or Giving USA. Nonetheless, this activity appeals to both

companies and nonprofits and may be a mutually satisfactory substitute for charitable giving.

- There is no practical reason why companies should use pretax income as the basis for determining their charitable contribution levels. There is no reason not to pursue a strategy in which charitable support to non-profits increases without consuming an increasing share of corporate profits.[17]

The Conference Board, which has surveyed the charitable giving behavior of firms, wrote that, in 1999, "companies reported that 28% of their contributions were in forms other than cash donations, the highest level of non-cash expenditures ever reported by companies in the Conference Board Analyses of cash and non-cash giving."[18] Among the industries reporting the largest non-cash percentages were "chemical companies, which donated 68% of their 1999 contributions in forms other than cash; pharmaceutical companies, with 64%; manufacturers of computer and office equipment, with 59%; printing, publishing and medical firms with 48%."[19] In a table of cash and non-cash contributions by industry, it was reported that the 10 companies in the Food/Beverage/Tobacco industrial classification gave 28% of their contributions in in-kind giving.[20]

An article which appeared in *Worth* magazine provided information on the 50 companies that gave the most in 1999. The table which follows is a subset of the five food concerns which appear in the complete listing of 50 companies.

Table 1. Charitable Giving by Food Concerns

Company	Cash Giving	In-Kind Giving	1999 Total Giving	Giving as % of Profit
Kroger	$43,600,000	$31,400,000	$75,000,000	11.8
Safeway	$27,000,000	$35,586,069	$62,586,069	6.5
General Mills	$30,912.124	$8,000,000	$38,912,124	6.3
Sara Lee	$19,732,000	$19,050,000	$38,782,000	3.3
Kellogg	$12,000,000	$21,742,648	$33,742,648	10.0

Several observations may be made by comparing the companies in table 1 with the statistics of the remaining 45 companies that made the largest charitable gifts. In general, giving by food companies as a percentage of profits is high. In table 1, it is shown that Sara Lee gave 3.3% of profits (the lowest percentage of the firms listed in the chart). According to the article in *Worth*, only four nonfood related companies gave a greater percentage of their profits than Sara Lee (Dupont; J.C. Penney; Target, and the United Parcel Service). All of the food companies showed substantial in-kind giving while 15 of the remaining 45 companies showed no in-kind giving at all. With the exceptions of Gannett and Dupont, all companies that provided greater in-kind giving than cash giving also benefit from the enhanced deduction provision in the Internal Revenue Code. Those companies are pharmaceutical/health care or computer/information technology firms.

Issues and Observations

Corporate charitable contributions are rarely a prominent issue in consideration of U.S. tax policy. First, corporate managers have been careful about making charitable contributions since their responsibility is to provide the highest rate of return that is legally possible to those who have invested in the corporation. Often, making charitable contributions conflicts with this mandate. Having said that, corporations do make charitable gifts all the time. It is also true that their contributions are usually intended to enhance the corporation's visibility or image before the consuming public. That is, goodwill is a valuable asset for a corporation, and charitable contributions help to create that goodwill. However, it generally makes no difference to a corporation whether it deducts its payment as a charitable contribution or as a business advertising expense because either deduction lowers its federal income tax by the same amount.[21] Only when the special rules for contributions of inventory come into play does it make a difference as to how the gift is viewed and how the value of the contribution changes under current tax law.

Equity Concerns

There are equity challenges to extending the current enhanced tax deduction for corporate contributions of food to all taxpayers engaged in a trade or business, such as small family farms and family operated restaurants (sometimes referred to as entrepreneurs in this report). A primary obstacle is that the cost basis could be higher for corporations than for a small business. This result can be caused by the inclusion of wages and germane taxes (such as Social Security, unemployment taxes, etc.) that are paid by corporations, but are not always included in the cost basis of small businesses such as farmers who grow crops or owner-chefs who own individual restaurants. Since it can be expected that (one-half of the) appreciation of the crops generally would be lower for corporations, with the full deductibility of the cost basis, than for individual farmers, an inherent advantage would still be given corporate farmers with their higher cost basis. For example, if a corporation has a cost basis of $7,000 with appreciation of $3,000, this equals a market price of $10,000. A small entrepreneur would more likely have a cost basis of $3,000 and an appreciation rate of $7,000 for the same $10,000 market price. In the corporate case, one-half of the appreciation ($1,500) and the cost basis ($7,000) is equal to $8,500. In the case of the entrepreneur, one half the appreciation ($3,500) plus the cost basis ($3,000) is equal to $6,500. Thus, the corporation would receive nearly $2,000 more in deductibility.

It can be argued that the temporary law provides more equity among all taxpayers engaged in a trade or business than the current, permanent law which provides the enhanced deduction only to C corporations and does not include provisions for S businesses or individuals.

Tax Rate Differentials

In addition, it should be noted that tax rates and the graduation of those rates are different for individuals and corporations. Current law provides for corporate tax rates which range between 15% and 35% depending on the company's taxable income (phase-outs can make the effective rates for certain corporations rise as high as 39%). In tax year 2005, individuals will be subject to six tax rates ranging from 10% to 35%. In all cases, whether corporate or individual, the value of the enhanced deduction is dependent on the applicable tax rate. Typically, those with higher incomes would receive more advantage than those with lower incomes under the proposal.[22] Thus, it does not appear that full equity can be achieved through the extension of the current enhanced deduction for corporate gifts of food inventory to all taxpayers engaged in a trade or business. For example, a large corporation will most likely have a 35% rate. A small farmer filing a joint return whose income is less than $182,800 would be subject to a 28% rate. It may also be noted that the law applies only to food inventory, and as such, may discriminate against other similar forms of charitable contributions (such as gifts of clothing for the poor).

An Alternative Possibility: Tax Credit

From an economic perspective, the use of a tax credit, rather than a deduction, would better promote equity among all business taxpayers. Tax deductions are useful in defining income that should be taxable. For instance, in the case of individuals, it is typically argued that charitable contributions are made using funds that are no longer within the taxpayer's control and, thus, monies to which the taxpayer may no longer lay real claim. In this instance, the deduction helps to define the income that should be subject to tax.

Tax credits are subtracted from tax liability, whereas tax deductions are subtracted from income to determine the amount subject to tax. The net result is that for each $1 of tax credit the tax liability is reduced by $1. Deductions reduce tax liability by only a percentage of the deduction, depending upon the tax rate of the taxpayer. Tax credits are used primarily to reduce taxes directly rather than to define the base on which taxes should be collected and are frequently used as incentives. Further, tax credits can be used by all eligible taxpayers (who owe taxes) since they are subtracted directly from tax liability.

Other Issues

We have assumed that farmers may donate crops to qualified organizations for gleaning, which is defined as the act of a tax-exempt organization that either harvests the crop or gathers the grain or other produce left in the field after an initial harvest.[23] A farmer's decision to abandon crops in the field is typically made at the time of harvest. Fixed costs such as seed, fertilizer, and other costs such as purchased irrigation water (typically referred to as sunk costs) are not taken into consideration when making the decision to harvest. The decision to move a crop to market is based on whether the farmer will receive a market price for the crop that exceeds his cost for harvesting, packing and transporting the crop. In those cases where the decision is marginal (i.e., the point at which the farmer may break even) to harvest or not to harvest, it would be to the farmer's advantage to make use of the proposed enhanced deduction. By opting to have the crop gleaned by an exempt organization, no expenses associated with the harvest would be incurred, while a deduction would be available to offset taxation of the farmer's other taxable funds. Alternatively, the use of a carryover of the deduction for offsetting taxable funds could be available for up to five future tax years.

Appropriate Valuation of Donated Goods

A primary problem with products that have shelf lives is determining an appropriate value for the goods donated. Under certain proposals, the fair market value can be determined by the price of the same or similar food items sold by the taxpayer at the time of the contribution (or, sold in the recent past). Prior legislative language provided a safe harbor for taxpayers by defining "apparently wholesome food" that is eligible for donation. Under this proposed definition, the food may be apparently wholesome even if it is not readily marketable "due to appearance, age, freshness, grade, size, surplus, or other conditions." This definition is the same as provided in the *Bill Emerson Good Samaritan Food Donation Act*.[24]

In discussing this valuation problem, which is now a part of the legislative history,[25] a court case was cited where the Tax Court held the value of surplus bread inventory donated to a qualified charity was determined to be the same as the full retail price of the bread.[26] The Internal Revenue Service (IRS) contended that the retail value of the bread was half the normal sales price since the industry practice of major bakers is to discount four-day-old bread.[27] If the court had ruled the value of the bread was half the retail selling price (following industry practice), then Lucky Stores would have received no tax benefit and, thus, no encouragement to make such charitable donations.[28] The court's findings contradicted regulations issued by IRS.

One effect of passage of the proposed legislation would be to make the ruling in the *Lucky Stores* case the law of the land rather than being applicable only in the 9th Circuit. Opponents of the provision may argue that there are economic incentives (rather than tax incentives) for stores to continue to make such gifts. For example, there are costs associated with disposal of product.[29] Obviously, the gifting of products reduces disposal costs. In addition, companies can expect goodwill (commonly referred to as "cause marketing"). High profile contributions can contribute to image building for the firm and influence public opinion.[30]

It is anticipated that opponents of the legislation may argue that the changes would reduce revenues to the federal government. The Joint Committee on Taxation estimated that enactment of the provision in the "Care" legislation introduced during the 108th Congress would have resulted in a revenue loss of $255 million over the five-year period of 2002-2006, with an estimated increase to $626 million over the 10-year period of 2002-2011.[31] It was expected that other industries would have requested similar tax treatment,[32] which, if granted, would have lead to an additional reduction in tax receipts at a time of increasing budget deficits.

Direct Subsidy Programs as an Alternative

In the past, some have argued that it would be preferable for the government to pay directly for the additional support of food programs rather than creating expenditures through the tax system. Direct government subsidies would assure that such funds were likely to be allocated under objective procedures and would, therefore, go to all the poor strictly based on need. Further, it is argued that a direct government spending program would assure that expenditures would be subjected to periodic review under the budgetary process.

Some feel that the expansion of the charitable deduction to all taxpayers engaged in a trade or business provides greater (food) benefits to people living near farm production areas where the food is harvested, more so than to people living far from farm areas in large cities. Further, gifts made by farms are likely to be seasonal. Others note that more restaurants are located in populated areas and that they may be the primary beneficiaries of the provision. Proponents of the proposals are most likely to argue that more food would be available to the elderly, poor, and infants for each tax expenditure dollar than through other direct government food expenditure programs. Another argued advantage would be that, most likely, there would be minimal federal government involvement in administering the program. Both sides have agreed that the proposed change would add complexity to the tax return filing process for a greater number of taxpayers in the charitable contribution arena. Some have suggested that since there is a sunset provision Congress would have an opportunity to evaluate the success of the change.

REFERENCES

[1] U.S. Congress, Committee on Homeland Security and Governmental Affairs, S.Rept. 110-338, Federal Food Donation Act of 2008 (S. 2420), May 22, 2008.
[2] Churches are not required to file for certification with the Internal Revenue Service.
[3] The Internal Revenue Code normally subjects corporate profits to the corporate income tax under its subchapter C; corporations subject to income tax are thus often referred to as "C corporations."
[4] S corporations are not subject to the corporate income tax and their net profits are passed through to the individual shareholders, the number of which must be limited to 75 or less, who are taxed on the profits under the individual income tax.
[5] The definition provides for (1) stock in trade of the taxpayer or other property of a kind which would properly be included in the inventory of the taxpayer if on hand at the close of the taxable year, or property held by the taxpayer primarily for sale to customers in the ordinary course of his trade or business; (2) property, used in his trade or business, of a character which is subject to the allowance for depreciation provided in section 167, or real property used in his trade or business. Examples would be dented canned goods given by Safeway to a food bank, Sara Lee frozen goods given to a homeless women's shelter, or contributions of cereal by General Mills to Second Harvest.
[6] The Internal Revenue Code provides that "the use of the property by the donee is related to the purpose or function constituting the basis for its exemption under section 501."
[7] Internal Revenue Code § 170(e)(3)(i).
[8] Internal Revenue Code §170(e)(3)(ii).
[9] Internal Revenue Code §170(e)(3)(iii).
[10] Internal Revenue Code §170(e)(3)(iiii).
[11] Lucky Stores, Inc. v. Commissioner, 105 T.C. 420 (1995).
[12] Since one-half the fair market value was less than basis, the donor would have received the exact same deduction for a contribution to a food bank or for discarded inventory which, in both cases, is a tax deduction for basis.
[13] No deduction is to be allowed for any part of the unrealized appreciation which would have been ordinary income (if the property had been sold) because of the application of the recapture provisions relating to depreciation. Also, no deduction is allowed for certain mining exploration expenditures, certain excess farm losses,

certain soil and water conservation expenditures, and certain land-clearing expenditures.

[14] U.S. Congress, Joint Committee on Taxation, *Summary of the Tax Reform Act of 1976 (H.R. 10612, 94th Congress. P.L. 94-455)*, committee print, 94th Cong., 2nd sess., December 29, 1976, (Washington: GPO, 1976), p. 673.

[15] Ibid. p. 673.

[16] *Giving USA 2004, The Annual Report on Philanthropy for the Year 2006.* A publication of the Giving USA Foundation, researched and written by the Center on Philanthropy at Indiana University, (Glenview, IL, 2007) p. 100.

[17] Ann E. Kaplan, ed. *Giving USA 1998, The Annual Report on Philanthropy for the Year 1997.* American Association of Fund-Raising Counsel Trust for Philanthropy. (New York, 1998), p. 22.

[18] Audris D. Tillman. *Corporate Contributions in 1999.* The Conference Board, Inc., Research Report 1284-00-RR, New York, 2000, p. 15.

[19] Ibid.

[20] Ibid. p. 16.

[21] Also, note that charitable contributions may not exceed certain levels. In the case of corporations it is 10%. For individuals, the limitation is generally 50%.

[22] The graduated corporate tax rates both increase and decrease across taxable incomes. This graduation is justified as an aid to small businesses. As corporate taxable income rises, the graduation is eliminated through phase-outs. Corporate tax rates for taxable income up to $50,000 are 15%; between $50K and $75K the rate is 25%; between $75K and $ 100K the rate is 34%; between $ 100K and $335K the rate is 39%; between $335K and $10M the rate is 34%; between $10M and $15M the rate is 35%; between $15M and $18,333,333 the rate is 38%; taxable incomes over that amount pay at the 35% rate. Most very large corporations pay a tax rate of 35%.

[23] Proposed legislation is silent on this topic.

[24] 42 U.S.C.A. § 1791 (Bill Emerson Good Samaritan Food Donation Act).

[25] U.S. Congress, Joint Committee on Taxation, *Description of an Amendment in the Nature of a Substitute to H.R. 7, the "Community Solutions Act of 2001,"* committee print, 107th Cong., 1st sess. (Washington: GPO, 2001), p. 10.

[26] Lucky Stores, Inc. v. Commissioner, 105 T.C. 420 (1995).

[27] The Court ruled that Lucky Stores sold four-day old bread at full retail price and did not discount sales to its own customers. Further, the Court found that the quantity of sales of four-day old bread was irrelevant. The Court noted that the IRS argument over the "industry practice" of discounting four-day old bread did not prove fair market value but, rather, that Lucky Stores could have sold the bread at a discount if it so chose to do so.

[28] [28] Since one-half the fair market value was less than basis, Lucky Stores would have received the exact same deduction for a contribution to a food bank or for discarded inventory which, in both cases, is a tax deduction for basis.

[29] Some products have higher disposal costs than others. For example, unneeded medical supplies and certain computer components may have high destruction costs.

[30] It should be noted that Lucky Stores deliberately overproduced bread. By doing so they were able to assure that bread was in stock at all times for customer needs. Thus, they were able to keep their customers happy (and in their stores to purchase product) while also knowing that they would receive a tax benefit for the overproduction. Often

when a firm has excess capacity, an additional unit's cost may be relatively small because there are many fixed costs. Or in some cases, there may be fixed costs associated with goods produced for sale rather than goods produced for contributions (such as the expenses associated with advertising costs for goods sold).

[31] Cost estimates for the proposals introduced in the 109th Congress are not available.

[32] As an example, the pharmaceutical industry could request a similar safe harbor for valuing drugs donated near their expiration date.

In: Hunger in America: Issues and Assistance
Editor: Gaston T. LaBue, pp. 81-117
ISBN: 978-1-60692-803-5

Chapter 4

FOOD STAMP PROGRAM: USE OF ALTERNATIVE METHODS TO APPLY FOR AND MAINTAIN BENEFITS COULD BE ENHANCED BY ADDITIONAL EVALUATION AND INFORMATION ON PROMISING PRACTICES*

United States Government Accountability Office

WHAT GAO FOUND

All states use mail and about half of states use or have begun developing online services and call centers to provide access to the food stamp program. Almost all states allow households to submit applications, report changes, and submit recertifications through the mail, and 26 states have implemented or are developing systems for households to perform these tasks on-line. Almost half of the states are using or developing call centers and states also are allowing households to participate in telephone interviews instead of an in-office interview. States have taken a variety of actions to help households use on-line services and call centers, such as sending informational mailings, holding community meetings, and using community partners.

Insufficient information is available to determine the results of using alternative methods. Few evaluations have been conducted identifying the effect of alternative methods on program access, decision accuracy, or administrative costs. Evaluating the effectiveness of alternative methods is challenging in part because limited data are available, states are using a combination of methods, and studies can be costly to conduct. Federal and state officials reported that while they believe alternative methods can help households in several ways, such as increasing flexibility and efficiency in the application process, certain types of households may have difficulty using or accessing alternative methods. In addition, technology and staffing challenges may hinder the use of alternative methods.

---

* Excerpted from GAO Report GAO-07-573, dated May 2007.

To maintain program integrity while implementing alternative methods, the states GAO reviewed used a variety of strategies, such as using software to verify the information households submit, communicating with other states to detect fraud, or using finger imaging. Although there has been some concern that without frequent in-person interaction with caseworkers, households may not submit required documents on time and thus be denied benefits on procedural grounds ("procedural denials"), GAO's limited analysis of FNS data found no considerable fluctuations in the rate of procedural denials in the five states between fiscal years 2000 and 2005. The states GAO reviewed have instituted several approaches to prevent procedural denials.

Why GAO Did this Study

One in 12 Americans participates in the federal Food Stamp Program, administered by the Food and Nutrition Service (FNS). States have begun offering individuals alternatives to visiting the local assistance office to apply for and maintain benefits, such as mail-in procedures, call centers, and online services. GAO was asked to examine: (1) what alternative methods states are using to increase program access; (2) what is known about the results of these methods, particularly on program access for target groups, decision accuracy, and administrative costs; and (3) what actions states have taken to maintain program integrity while implementing alternative methods. GAO surveyed state food stamp administrators, reviewed five states in depth, analyzed FNS data and reports, and interviewed program officials and stakeholders.

What GAO Recommends

GAO recommends that the Secretary of Agriculture direct FNS to (1) work with the Economic Research Service (ERS) to enhance their research agendas to include projects that would determine the effects of alternative methods; (2) conduct analyses of data received from states implementing waivers or demonstration projects waiving the face-to-face interview; and (3) disseminate and regularly update information on promising practices states are using to implement alternative methods. FNS and ERS generally agreed with GAO's findings, conclusions, and recommendations.

Abbreviations

EBT	Electronic Benefits Transfer
ERS	Economic Research Service
FNS	Food and Nutrition Service
FSP	Food Stamp Program
PRWORA	Personal Responsibility and Work Opportunity Reconciliation Act of 1996
QC	quality control

SSI	Supplemental Security Income
TANF	Temporary Assistance for Needy Families
USDA	U.S. Department of Agriculture

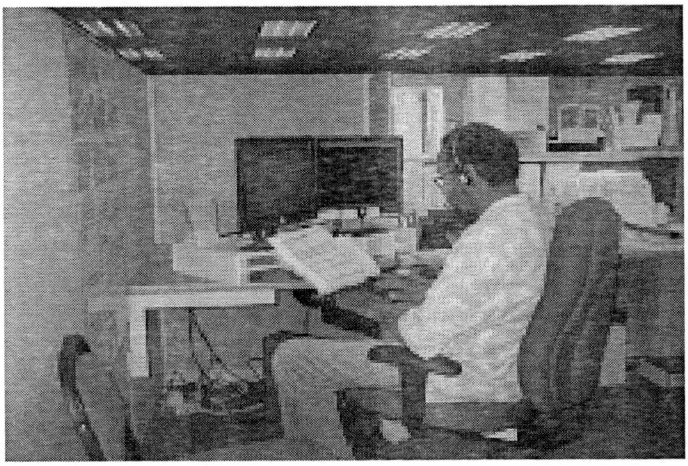

Source: GAO.

May 3, 2007
The Honorable Tom Harkin
Chairman

Committee on Agriculture, Nutrition, and Forestry
United States Senate

Dear Mr. Chairman:

Almost 1 in every 12 Americans participates in the federal Food Stamp Program, which helps low-income individuals and families purchase nutritious food, such as meat, dairy products, fruits, and vegetables. In fiscal year 2005, the program, jointly administered by the U.S. Department of Agriculture's (USDA) Food and Nutrition Service (FNS) and the states, provided about $29 billion in benefits to nearly 26 million people, about half of whom were children.[1]

Although participation in the program has increased substantially in recent years, about 40 percent of people who were eligible for the program did not participate in 2004, the most recent year data are available. Elderly individuals, non-citizens that may have limited English proficiency, and working families have consistently participated at lower rates than the eligible population as a whole and FNS has targeted these subgroups to increase participation. Even though there are many reasons people may not participate in the program, some research has shown that the administrative burden of applying for and maintaining eligibility for benefits may be a factor, particularly for people who are elderly or who work during the hours local public assistance offices are open. Participation in the program generally requires individuals to submit an application, participate in an interview at initial application and at least annually, provide verification of certain information, report certain changes in household circumstances while receiving benefits, and reapply for benefits at the end of the certification period (recertification). While completing the Food Stamp

Program application and recertification process has traditionally involved visiting the local assistance office in person for interviews or to submit applications and other documentation, states have begun offering alternatives in the last several years, such as mail-in procedures, call centers, and on-line services.

While FNS has allowed states to adopt these new ways of accessing the program, it also has a quality control system in place to monitor program integrity. Under this system, FNS monitors decision accuracy, including how accurately states determine food stamp eligibility and calculate benefits. In addition to monitoring the payment error rate, FNS estimates the rate of cases denied, suspended, or terminated incorrectly, which is called the negative error rate. FNS and USDA's Economic Research Service (ERS) also fund Food Stamp Program research.

To understand what alternative approaches states are using to help households apply for and maintain benefits and what is known about the results of using these methods, we examined: (1) the alternative methods to the traditional application and recertification process states are using to increase program access; (2) what is known about the results of these methods, particularly on program access for target groups, decision accuracy, and administrative costs; and (3) what actions states have taken to maintain program integrity while implementing alternative methods.

To answer these questions, we surveyed food stamp administrators in the 50 states and the District of Columbia[2] to collect information on what alternative methods states are using or planning to use (mail, call centers, on-line services), how performance of these methods is measured, and what is known about the results of using these methods. To augment information from our state survey, we conducted four site visits (Florida, Texas, Utah, and Washington) and one set of semi-structured telephone interviews (Pennsylvania). We selected states that have at least one FNS- approved waiver of the face-to-face interview requirement and reflect some variation in state participation rates. We also considered recommendations from FNS officials, advocacy group representatives, and researchers. For each of the five states we reviewed in depth, we interviewed state officials administering and developing policy for the Food Stamp Program, local officials in the assistance offices and call centers where services are provided, and representatives from community- based organizations that provide food assistance. We analyzed data provided by FNS and the states we reviewed in depth to provide background for our discussions with officials about state trends for specific measures (participation, payment accuracy, administrative costs, and reasons for denial). We also reviewed FNS reports and related studies. We held discussions with program stakeholders, including officials at FNS headquarters and regional offices, and representatives of advocacy organizations. Appendix I explains our methodology in more detail. We performed our work from September 2006 to March 2007 in accordance with generally accepted government auditing standards.

Results in Brief

All states use mail and about half of states use or have begun developing on-line services and call centers to provide access to the Food Stamp Program. Almost all states told us they allow households to submit applications, report changes, and submit recertifications through the mail, and 26 states have implemented or are developing systems to allow households to submit applications, report changes, or submit recertifications on-line. In addition, almost half of the states are using or developing call centers and states are also using flexibility authorized by FNS to increase use of the telephone as an alternative to visiting the local assistance office. For example, FNS has approved administrative waivers allowing 20 states to substitute a telephone interview for the face-to-face interview for all households at recertification without needing to document that coming into the office would be a hardship for the household. States have taken a variety of actions to help households use on-line services and call centers, such as sending informational mailings, holding community meetings, and employing call center staff who speak languages other than English. States are also relying on community-based organizations, such as food banks, to help households use alternative methods. For example, four of the five states we interviewed provide grants to community-based organizations to inform households about the program and help them complete the application process.

Insufficient information is available to determine the results of using alternative methods to provide access to the Food Stamp Program, but federal and state officials reported that despite some challenges, they believe these methods are making it easier for some households to access program benefits. Few evaluations have been conducted to identify the effect of alternative methods on program access, decision accuracy, or administrative costs. FNS has two studies under way that will describe implementation of alternative methods such as on-line services and call centers, but it is unlikely that these studies will use research approaches that would identify the effect of alternative methods. Further, while states reported monitoring the performance of call centers and on-line services, none of the states has conducted evaluations that would identify the effect of the alternative methods on program access, decision accuracy, or administrative costs. State officials reported implementing a combination of methods over time, making it difficult to isolate the effect of specific methods. Despite this, federal and state officials said that they believe that giving households alternatives to visiting the food stamp office can help improve access to benefits. For example, in the five states we reviewed in depth, officials and community partners said that allowing telephone interviews is especially beneficial for working families and the elderly because they reduce barriers from transportation, child care, or work responsibilities, as well as the stigma of visiting the assistance office. However, officials and community partners also said that certain types of households, such as those with limited English proficiency, the elderly, and those with mental disabilities, may have difficulty using on-line applications and navigating call center phone systems. The advantages of alternative methods to households also may depend on the technology and staff available. For example, on-line applications without electronic signature capability have limited benefit because households are required to also submit an actual signature through mail, fax, or in person. Further, inadequate numbers of staff and unskilled staff may limit the advantages of alternative methods because households may not be able to receive the information and assistance needed to successfully apply for or maintain benefits.

The five states we reviewed used a variety of strategies to maintain program integrity while implementing alternative methods, some of which were in place long before implementation of the alternative access methods. All five states used software to help with verification of household circumstances by, for example, matching state food stamp caseloads against wage reporting systems and other databases to identify unreported household income and assets. Nationwide, about half of the states participate in quarterly matches with other states to detect households receiving food stamp benefits in more than one state at a time. In addition, all five states we reviewed developed special caseworker training on topics such as how to detect misinformation provided by a household over the telephone. State and local food stamp officials told us they believed that using alternative methods had not increased the frequency of fraud and abuse in the program because the verification process is the same whether or not a worker sees an individual face-to-face. There has been some concern that without face-to-face contact with caseworkers, households may not know when or how to submit paperwork or complete other tasks and would thus be denied benefits on procedural grounds ("procedural denials"). However, our limited analysis of FNS data found no considerable fluctuations in the rate of procedural denials in the five states between fiscal years 2000 and 2005. To prevent improper procedural denials, the five states we reviewed instituted such approaches as reviewing case actions, correcting addresses for returned mail, and changing automated systems to prevent caseworkers from prematurely denying cases.

To improve USDA's ability to assess the effectiveness of its funded efforts, we are recommending that the Secretary of Agriculture: direct FNS and the Economic Research Service (ERS) to work together to enhance their research agendas to include projects that would determine the effect of alternative methods on program access, decision accuracy, and administrative costs of the Food Stamp Program; and direct FNS to conduct analyses of data received from states implementing waivers or demonstration projects waiving the face-to-face interview and require states implementing waivers or demonstration projects to collect and report data that would facilitate such analyses. Further, to help states implement alternative methods to provide access to the Food Stamp Program, we are recommending that FNS disseminate and regularly update information on states' implementation of alternative methods to the traditional application and recertification process. FNS and ERS generally agreed with our findings, conclusions, and recommendations and cited steps the agency is taking to monitor and evaluate state implementation of alternative access methods. FNS and ERS also provided technical comments, which were incorporated into the report as appropriate.

BACKGROUND

The federal Food Stamp Program is intended to help low-income individuals and families obtain a more nutritious diet by supplementing their income with benefits to purchase eligible foods at authorized food retailers, such as meat, dairy products, fruits, and vegetables, but not items such as soap, tobacco, or alcohol. FNS pays the full cost of food stamp benefits and shares the states' administrative costs—with FNS usually paying slightly less than 50 percent—and is responsible for promulgating program regulations and ensuring that state officials administer the program in compliance with program rules.[3] The states administer the program by determining whether households meet the program's eligibility requirements, calculating monthly benefits for qualified households, and issuing benefits to participants through an electronic benefits transfer system.

Program Participation

In fiscal year 2005, the Food Stamp Program issued almost $28.6 billion in benefits to about 25.7 million individuals per month, and the maximum monthly food stamp benefit for a household of four living in the continental United States in fiscal year 2007 was $518. As shown in figure 1, program participation decreased during the late 1990s, partly due to an improved economy, but rose again from 2000 to 2005. The number of food stamp recipients follows the trend in the number of people living at or below the federal poverty level.

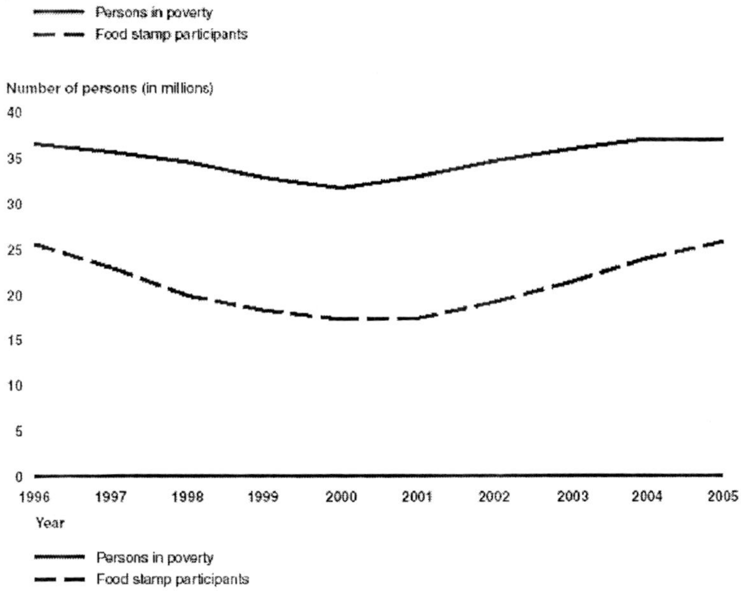

Source: GAO analysis of FNS and U.S. Census data.

Notes: Poverty data are by calendar year and participation data are by fiscal year.

Preliminary FNS data indicate that participation will continue to grow to nearly 27 million people receiving about $30 billion in food stamp benefits in fiscal year 2006.

Figure 1. Food Stamp Participation and Poverty Trends.

In addition to the economic growth in the late 1990s, another factor contributing to the decrease in number of participants from 1996 to 2001 was the passage of the Personal Responsibility and Work Opportunity Reconciliation Act of 1996 (PRWORA), which added work requirements and time limits to cash assistance and made certain groups ineligible to receive food stamp benefits. In some cases, this caused participants to believe they were no longer eligible for food stamps when TANF benefits were ended.[4] Since 2000, that downward trend has reversed, and experts believe that the downturn in the U.S. economy, coupled with changes in the Food Stamp Program's rules and administration, has led to an increase in the number of food stamp participants.

Determination of Eligibility and Benefits

Eligibility for participation in the Food Stamp Program is based primarily on a household's income and assets. To determine a household's eligibility, a caseworker must first determine the household's gross income, which cannot exceed 130 percent of the poverty level for that year as determined by the Department of Health and Human Services, and net income, which cannot exceed 100 percent of the poverty level (or about $1,799 per month for a family of three living in the continental United States in fiscal year 2007). Net income is determined by deducting from gross income a portion of expenses such as dependent care costs, medical expenses for elderly individuals, utilities costs, and housing expenses.

The Process of Applying for and Maintaining Benefits

The application process for the Food Stamp Program requires households to complete and submit an application to a local assistance office, participate in an interview, and submit documentation to verify household circumstances (see table 1). Applicants may need to make more than one visit to the assistance office to complete the application process. After eligibility is established, households are certified eligible for food stamps for periods ranging from 1 to 24 months, depending on household circumstances and state policy. While households are receiving benefits, they must report changes in household circumstances that may affect eligibility or benefit amounts. States may choose to require households to report changes within 10 days of occurrence (incident reporting) or at specified intervals (periodic reporting). States also have the option to adopt a simplified system, which further reduces the burden of periodic reporting by requiring households to report changes that happen during a certification period only when their income rises above 130 percent of the federal poverty level.[5] Once the certification period ends, households must reapply for benefits, at which time eligibility and benefit levels are redetermined. The recertification process is similar to the application process. Households can be denied benefits or have their benefits end at any point during the process if they are determined ineligible under program rules or for procedural reasons, such as missing a scheduled interview or failing to provide the required documentation.

Table 1. Process to Apply for and Maintain Food Stamp Benefits

Apply for benefits	While receiving benefits	Recertify for benefits
• Complete and submit application to assistance office	• Report changes in household circumstances—such as household composition, income, and expenses—that may affect eligibility or benefit amounts	• Complete and submit recertification application to assistance office
• Participate in an interview		• Participate in an interview at least annually
• Submit documentation to verify information provided in the a pplicationand interview		• Submit documentation to verify information provided in the applicationand interview

Source: GAO analysis of FNS information.

While applying for and maintaining food stamp benefits has traditionally involved visiting a local assistance office, states have the flexibility to give households alternatives to visiting the office, such as using the mail, the telephone, and on-line services to complete the certification and recertification process. Alternative methods may be used to support other programs, such as Medicaid or TANF, since some food stamp participants receive benefits from multiple programs. Figure 2 illustrates a traditional office-based system and how states can use a number of alternative methods to determine applicants' eligibility without requiring them to visit an assistance office.

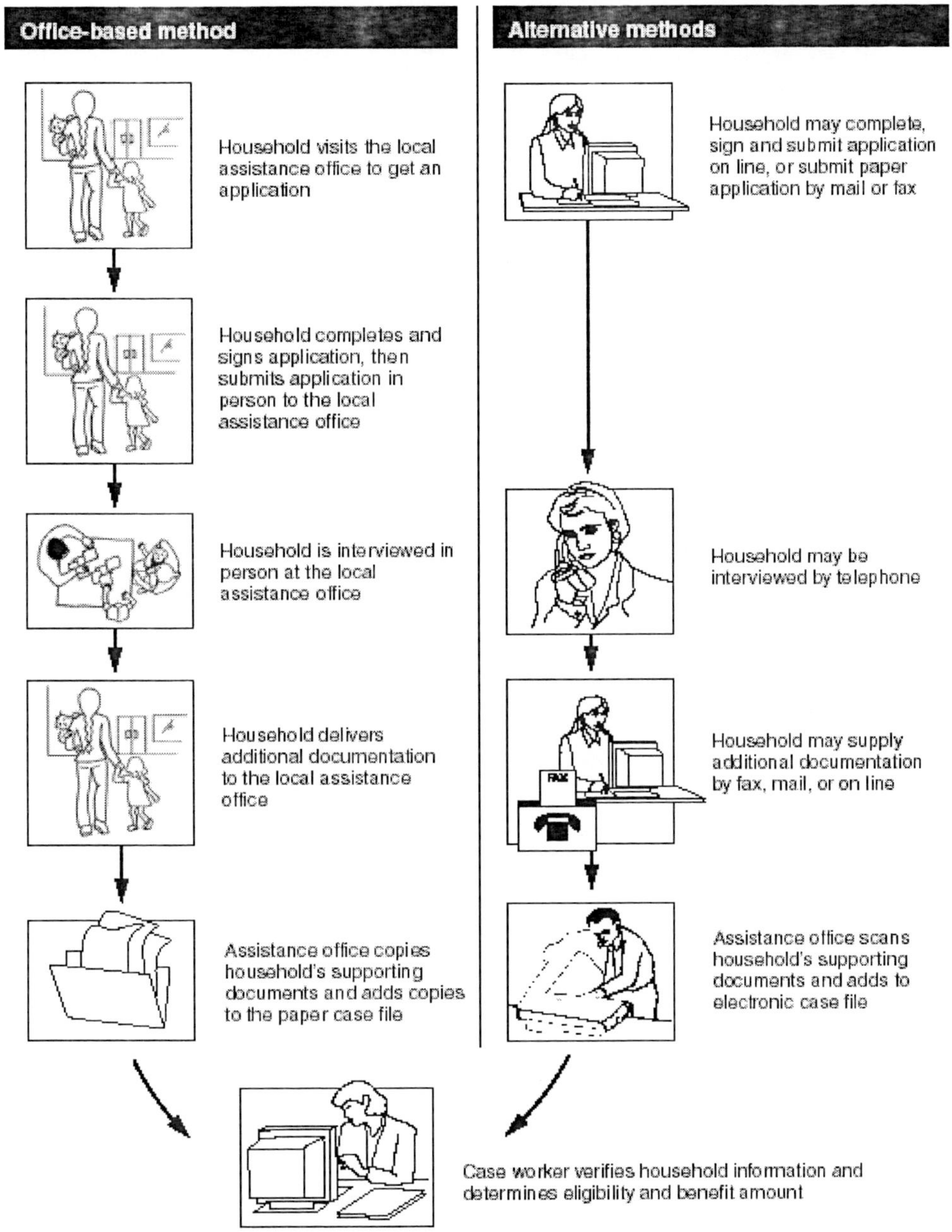

Source: GAO analysis.

Figure 2. Office-based Method Compared with Alternative Methods of Applying for Food Stamp Benefits.

Program Integrity

FNS and the states share responsibility for implementing a quality control system used to measure the accuracy of caseworker decisions concerning the amount of food stamp benefits households are eligible to receive and decisions to deny or end benefits. The food stamp payment error rate is calculated by FNS for the entire program, as well as every state, by adding overpayments (including payments higher than the amounts households are eligible for or payments to those who are not eligible for any benefit), and underpayments (payments lower than the amounts households are eligible for). The national payment error rate has declined by about 40 percent between 1999 and 2005, from 9.86 percent to a record low of 5.84 percent. FSP payment errors are caused primarily by caseworkers, usually when they fail to keep up with new information, and by participants when they fail to report needed information. Another type of error measured by FNS is the negative error rate, defined as the rate of cases denied, suspended, or terminated incorrectly. An example of incorrectly denying a case would be if a caseworker denied a household participation in the program because of excess income, but there was a calculation error and the household was actually eligible for benefits. FNS also monitors individual fraud and retailer trafficking of food stamp benefits.[6]

All States Use Mail and About Half of States Use or Have Begun Developing on- line Services and Call Centers to Provide Access to the Food Stamp Program

According to our survey, almost all states allow households to submit applications, report changes, and submit recertifications through the mail, and 26 states have implemented or are developing systems to allow households to perform these tasks on-line. Almost half of the states are using or developing call centers and states are also using flexibility authorized by FNS to increase use of the telephone as an alternative to visiting the local assistance office. States have taken a variety of actions to help households use on-line services and call centers, such as sending informational mailings, holding community meetings, and using community partners to assist households.

Almost All States Allow Households to Apply for Food Stamp Benefits and Maintain Eligibility by Mail and about Half of the States Are Using or Developing on-line Services

Many states are allowing households to apply for food stamp benefits, report changes in household circumstances, and complete recertification through the mail and on-line. [7]

- *Mail-In Procedures.* Results of our survey show that households can submit applications through the mail in all states, report changes through the mail in all but 1 state, and submit recertifications through the mail in 46 states. For example, Washington state officials told us that the recertification process involves mailing a recertification application package to households that they can mail back without visiting a local assistance office.
- *On-line Services.* All states we surveyed reported having a food stamp application available for households to download from a state website, as required by federal law, and 26 states (51 percent) have implemented or are developing Web-based systems in which households can submit initial applications, report changes, or submit

recertifications on line (see fig. 3). Most on-line applications were made available statewide and implemented within the last 3 years and states developing on-line services plan to implement these services within the next 2 years. All of the 14 states that reported currently providing online services allow households to submit initial food stamp applications on-line, but only 6 states allow households to report changes and 5 states allow households to complete recertification on- line.[8] Of the 14 states that reported using on-line applications, 2 reported they were only available in certain areas of the state. Only two states (Florida and Kansas) reported in our survey that the state closed program offices or reduced staff as a result of implementing on-line services.

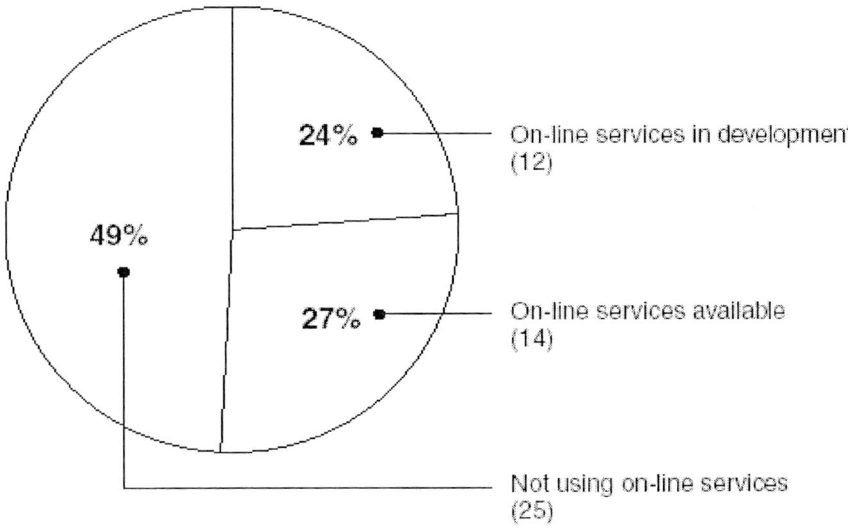

Source: GAO survey.

Figure 3. Number and Percentage of States Making On-line Services Available to Food Stamp Households.

Almost Half of States Are Using or Developing Call Centers and Using Telephone Interviews as an Alternative to Visiting the Local Assistance Office

Many states are using call centers, telephone interviews, or other technologies to help households access food stamp benefits or information without visiting a local assistance office.

- *Call Centers.* Nineteen states (37 percent) have made call centers available to households and an additional 4 states (8 percent) have begun development of call centers that will be available to households in 2007 (see fig. 4). Households have been able to use call centers in seven states for more than 3 years. Of the 19 states using call centers, 10 reported that call centers were only available in certain areas of the state. Only two states (Texas and Idaho) reported using private contractors to operate the call centers, but Texas announced in March 2007 that it was terminating its agreement with the private contractor (see fig. 10 for more details). FNS officials told us that the Idaho private call center provides general food stamp program information to callers, while inquiries about specific cases are transferred to state caseworkers. Indiana reported in our survey that the state plans to pilot call centers in certain areas of the state in August 2007 using a private contractor and complete a statewide transition in March 2008. Only two states (Florida and Arizona) reported in our survey that the state closed offices or reduced staff as a result of implementing call centers.

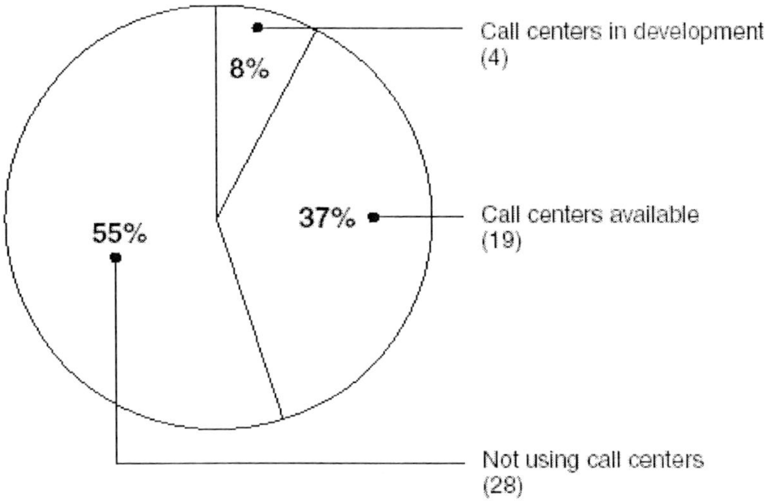

Source: GAO survey.

Figure 4. Number and Percentage of States Making Call Centers Available to Food Stamp Households.

Most states with call centers reported that households can use them to report changes in household circumstances, request a food stamp application and receive assistance filling it out, receive information about their case, or receive referrals to other programs. Only four states reported using their call centers to conduct telephone interviews. For example, local officials in Washington told us that households use their call center primarily to request information, report changes in household circumstances, and request an interview. Telephone interviews are conducted by caseworkers in the local assistance office.

- *Telephone Interviews.* Many states are using the flexibility provided by FNS to increase the use of the telephone as an alternative to households visiting the local assistance office. For example, FNS has approved administrative waivers for 20 states that allow states to substitute a telephone interview for the face-to-face interview for all households at recertification without documenting that visiting the assistance office would be a hardship for the household.[9] In addition to making it easier on households, this flexibility can reduce the administrative burden on the state to document hardship. FNS also allows certain states implementing demonstration projects to waive the interview requirement altogether for certain households. States we reviewed varied in terms of the proportion of interviews conducted over the phone. For example, Florida state and local officials estimated that about 90 percent of the interviews conducted in the state are completed over the telephone. Washington state officials estimated that 10 percent of application interviews and 30 percent of recertification interviews are conducted by phone. Table 2 describes the types of flexibility available to states and how many are taking advantage of each.

Table 2. Administrative Flexibility Available to States to Waive the Face-to-Face Interview

Description of flexibility	Availability	Year available or first approved by FNS	Number of statesd
Hardship policy Substitute telephone interview for face-to-face interview at application or recertification for all households experiencing a hardship as determined by the state. Hardship must be documented in the case file.	All states	1978	All states
Waiver at recertification Substitute telephone interview for face-to-face interview for all households at recertification without documenting hardship.	States with waivers	1992	20
Waiver at initial certificationb Substitute telephone interview for face-to-face interview for all households at initial certification without documenting hardship.	States with waivers	2005	3
Combined Application Projectsc Households can apply for food stamps at the same time they apply for or are recertified for Supplemental Security Income (SSI) with the Social Security Administration. Households are not required to have a separate interview to apply for food stamps.	States with demonstration projects	1995	• 10 have implemented • 6 approved or pending approval but have not implemented • 5 more have been invited to submit proposals
Elderly/Disabled Demonstration Projects Simplify the application process for elderly and/or disabled households in part by waiving the interview altogether.		2002	2

Source: GAO analysis of FNS information.

[a] These hardship conditions include, but are not limited to: illness, transportation difficulties, care of a household member, hardships due to residency in a rural area, prolonged severe weather conditions, or work or training hours that prevent the household from participating in an in-office interview. States must document hardship. The regulations also allow states to opt to substitute telephone interviews for face-to-face interviews for all households that have no earned income and in which all members are elderly or disabled.

[b] Limited to no more than 50 percent of the statewide caseload.

[c] The Food Stamp Act of 1977 included several access provisions, such as addressing the use of mail, telephone, or home visits for certification and joint food stamps and SSI application processing. Since 1986, federal law has required that applicants for or recipients of SSI must be informed of the opportunity to file a food stamp application at the SSA office when applying for SSI.

[d] See appendix II for specific state information.

- *Other Technologies.* Some states reported implementing other technologies that support program access. Specifically, according to our survey, 11 states (21 percent) have

alternative methods on food stamp program access, decision accuracy, or administrative costs. Although states monitor the implementation of alternative methods, isolating the effects of specific methods is difficult, in part because states typically have implemented a combination of methods over time. Despite the limited information on the effectiveness of alternative methods, federal and state officials believe that these methods can help many households by making it easier for them to complete the application or recertification process. However, technology and staffing challenges can hinder the use of these methods.

Few Evaluations Have Been Conducted and Determining the Effectiveness of Specific Methods Can Be Difficult

Few federal or state evaluations have been conducted to identify how using alternative methods, such as on-line applications or call centers, affects access to the Food Stamp Program, the accuracy of caseworker decisions about eligibility and benefit amounts, or administrative costs. Few evaluations have been conducted in part because evaluating the effectiveness of alternative methods is challenging, given that limited data are available, states are using a combination of methods, and studies can be costly to conduct.

Federal Evaluation and Monitoring

FNS and ERS have funded studies related to improving Food Stamp Program access, but none of these previous studies provide a conclusive assessment of the effectiveness of alternative methods and the factors that contribute to their success (see app. I for a list of the studies we selected and reviewed). Although these studies aimed to evaluate local office practices, grants, and demonstration projects, the methodological limitations of this research prevent assessments about the effectiveness of these efforts. An evaluation of the Elderly Nutrition Demonstration projects used a pre-post comparison group design to estimate the impact of the projects and found that food stamp participation among the elderly can be increased.[11] Two of the projects evaluated focused on making the application process easier by providing application assistance and simplifying the process, in part by waiving the interview requirement. However, one of the drawbacks of this study is that its findings are based on a small number of demonstrations, which affects the generalizability of the findings.

Two related FNS-funded evaluations are also under way, but it is unlikely these studies will identify the effects of using alternative methods.[12]

- An implementation study of Florida's efforts to modernize its system using call centers and on-line services involves a descriptive case study to be published in late summer 2007, incorporating both qualitative and quantitative data. The objectives of the study are to: describe changes to food stamp policies and procedures that have been made in support of modernization; identify how technology is used to support the range of food stamp eligibility determination and case management functions; and describe the experiences of food stamp participants, eligible non-participants, state food stamp staff, vendors, and community partners. This study will describe Florida's Food Stamp Program performance over time in comparison to the nation, other states in the region, and other large states. Performance data that will be reviewed includes program participation in general and by subgroup, timeliness of application processing, payment error rates, and administrative costs. However, the study will not isolate the effect of the modernization efforts on program performance.

- A national study of state efforts to enhance food stamp certification and modernize the food stamp program involves a state survey and case studies of 14 states and will result in a site visit report in late summer 2007, a comprehensive report in March 2009, and a public-use database systematically describing modernization efforts across all the states in May 2009. The national study will focus on four types of modernization efforts: policy changes to modernize FSP application, case management, and recertification procedures; reengineering of administrative functions; increased or enhanced use of technology; and partnering arrangements with businesses and nonprofit organizations. The goals of the study include documenting outcomes associated with food stamp modernization and examining the effect of these modernization efforts on four types of outcomes: program access, administrative cost, program integrity, and customer services. This study will compare performance data from the case study states with data from similar states and the nation as a whole, however, this analysis will not determine whether certain modernization efforts caused changes in performance.

USDA has also awarded $5 million in fiscal year 2006 to 5 grantees in Virginia, California, Georgia and Alabama to help increase access to the program, but there is currently no plan to publish an evaluation of the outcomes of these projects. The participation grants focus on efforts to simplify the application process and eligibility systems and each grantee plans to implement strategies to improve customer service by allowing Web-based applications and developing application sites outside the traditional social services office. Grantees are required to submit quarterly progress reports and final reports including a description of project activities and implementation issues.

Although few evaluations have been conducted, FNS monitors state and local offices and tracks state implementation of alternative methods to improve program access. FNS also collects and monitors data from states, such as the number of participants, amount of benefits issued, participation rates overall and by subgroup, timeliness of application processing, payment errors, negative errors, and administrative costs. FNS regional offices conduct program access reviews of selected local offices in all states to determine whether state and/or local policies and procedures served to discourage households from applying for food stamps or whether local offices had adopted practices to improve customer service. FNS also monitors major changes to food stamp systems using a process where FNS officials review and approve plans submitted by states related to system development and implementation, including major upgrades. States like Texas, Florida, and Indiana that have implemented major changes to their food stamp system, such as moving from a local assistance office service delivery model to call centers and online services, have worked with FNS through this process. Figure 7 describes FNS's monitoring of Indiana's plan to implement alternative access methods.

FNS has approved Indiana's plan to begin piloting a new eligibility system, including on-line services, call centers, and document management/imaging system with electronic case records in August 2007, and to implement the system statewide in March 2008. The state plans to outsource to a private contractor the responsibility for collecting application data and verification documents and processing reported changes. The plan includes keeping local assistance offices open in every county and transitioning most of the Indiana Family and Social Services Administration employees to work for the private contractor.

FNS is requiring the state agency to monitor the implementation and operation of the system and FNS plans to conduct on-site visits and review available data to monitor operations. FNS has requested that Indiana submit to them monthly reports and provided suggested reporting elements, but did not require the state to provide any particular data. Examples of the suggested data elements include: total applications filed, the disposition of cases, and amount of benefits authorized. FNS has requested that the state also report on monthly performance as compared to the corresponding period in the previous year. Because FNS has not required the state to submit certain data to them, it is not known at this time what information will be available or how it will be used to evaluate the performance of the state's new system.

Source: GAO analysis.

Figure 7. FNS Monitoring of Indiana's Plan to Implement Alternative Access Methods.

FNS has also encouraged states to share information about their efforts to increase access among states, but states reported needing additional opportunities to share information. FNS has funded national and regional conferences, travel by state officials to visit other states to learn about their practices, as well as provided states a guide to promising practices for improving program access.[13] The guide contains information about the goal of each practice, the number of places where the practice is in use, and contact information for a person in these offices. However, this guide has not been updated since 2002 and, for the most part, does not include any evidence that these efforts were successful or any lessons that were learned from these or other efforts.[14] In 2004, in response to recommendations from our prior report,[15] FNS compiled and posted 19 practices aimed to improve access from 11 states. FNS also has a form available on its website where states can submit promising practices to improve access, but to date, practices from this effort have not been published. In our survey, 13 states (about 25 percent) reported needing additional conferences or meetings with other states to share information.

State Evaluation and Monitoring

States also report monitoring use of alternative methods in the Food Stamp Program, but have not conducted evaluations of their effectiveness. In our survey, states reported monitoring several aspects of the performance of on-line services. As shown in figure 8, states most commonly used the number of applications submitted, the number of applications terminated before completion, and customer satisfaction to monitor the performance of on-line services. For example, Pennsylvania state officials monitor performance of their on-line system and meet regularly with community partners that help households submit applications for benefits to obtain feedback on how they can improve the system. Florida state officials told us they use responses to on-line feedback surveys submitted at the end of the on-line application to assess customer satisfaction with the state's on-line services.

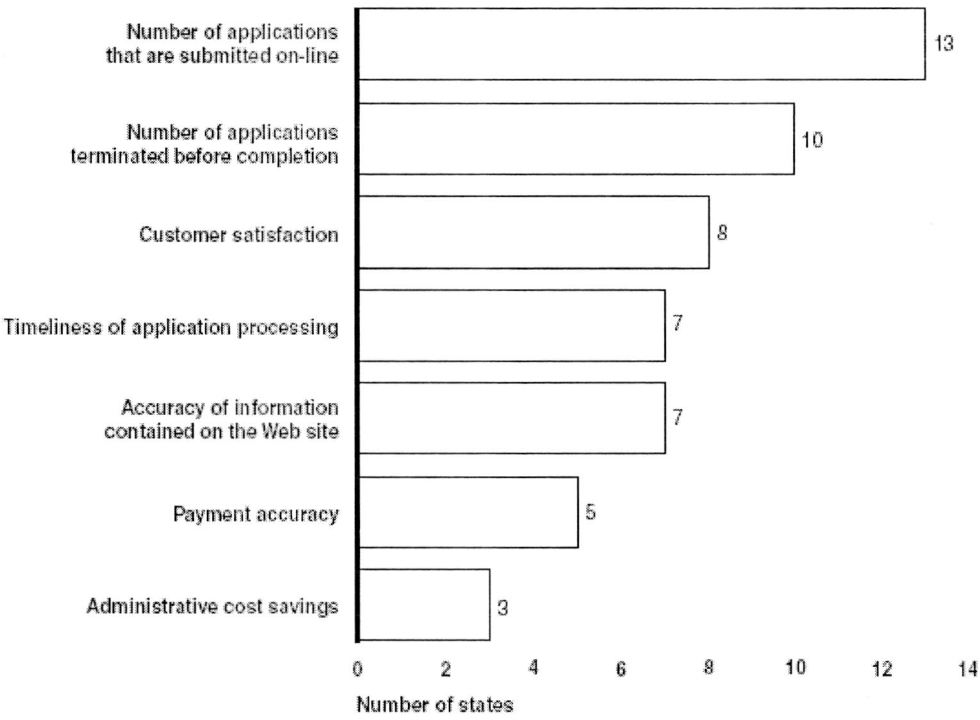

Source: GAO survey.

Figure 8. States' Use of Measures to Monitor Performance of On-line Services.

States also reported in our survey monitoring several aspects of the performance of their call centers. As shown in figure 9, most states with call centers reported monitoring the volume of transactions and calls to the center, customer satisfaction, the rate of abandoned calls, and the length of time callers are on hold before speaking with a caseworker. For example, Utah officials monitor several measures and added additional staff to the call center after observing increased hold times when they were implementing the call center to serve the Salt Lake City area. In addition, Washington state officials told us that they monitor call centers on an hourly basis, allowing call center managers to quickly increase the number of staff answering phones as call volumes increase.

Despite these monitoring efforts, no states reported conducting an evaluation of the effectiveness of on-line services in our survey and only one state reported conducting such an evaluation of its call centers. The report Illinois provided on its call center described customer and worker feedback on the performance of the call center, but did not provide a conclusive assessment of its effectiveness. Seven states implementing Combined Application Projects (CAP)[16] have submitted reports to FNS including data on the number of participants in the CAP project compared with when the project began, but do not use methods to isolate the effect of the project or determine whether participation by SSI recipients would have increased in the absence of the project. Two of the five states we reviewed said they planned to conduct reviews of their system. For example, Washington is conducting an internal quality improvement review of its call centers. It will compare call center operations with industry best practices and promising new technologies, and will identify the costs, services offered, and best practices used by the call centers.

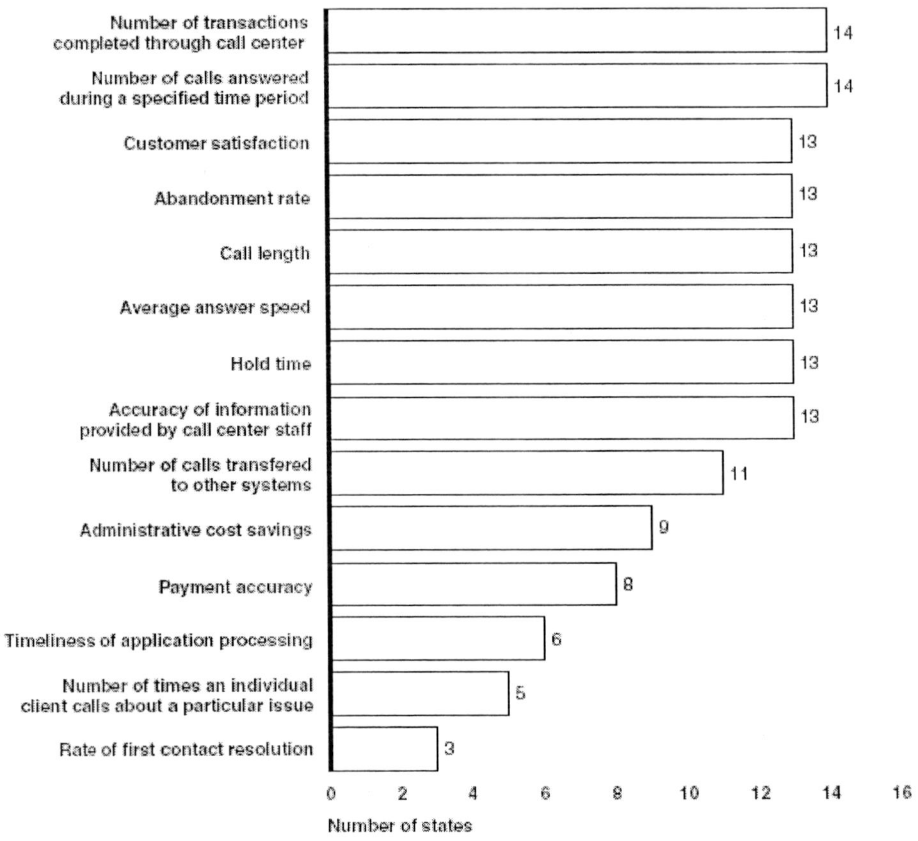

Source: GAO survey.

Figure 9. States' Use of Measures to Monitor Performance of Call Centers.

Evaluation Challenges

Few evaluations have been conducted, in part because evaluating the effectiveness of alternative methods is challenging. For example, states are limited in their ability to determine whether certain groups of households are able to use alternative methods because few states collect demographic information on households that use their on-line services and call centers. Only six states reported in our survey that they collect demographic information on the households that use on-line services and four states reported collecting demographic information on the households that use call centers. In addition, although FNS is requiring states with waivers to the face-to-face interview to track the payment accuracy of cases covered by these waivers, FNS has not yet assessed the effects of these methods on decision accuracy because it has not collected enough years of data to conduct reliable analyses of trends. Further, evaluations that isolate the effect of specific methods can be challenging because states implement methods at different times and are using a combination of methods. For example, Washington state implemented call centers in 2000, an on-line application and CAP in 2001, and document imaging and a waiver of the face-to-face interview at recertification in 2003. Sophisticated methodologies often are required to isolate the effects of certain practices or technologies. These studies can be costly to conduct because the data collection and analysis can take years to complete. For example, the two studies that we reviewed that aimed to isolate the effects of specific projects each cost over $1 million and were conducted over more than 3 years. Although evaluating the effects of alternative methods is challenging, FNS is collecting data from states through the waiver process that could be analyzed and previous ERSfunded studies have used methodologies that enable researchers to identify the effect of certain projects or practices on program access.

Federal and State Officials Report Alternative Methods Help Some Households Access Food Stamp Benefits, but Technology and Staffing Can Present Challenges

Despite the limited information on the effects of alternative methods, federal and state officials report that alternative methods, such as the availability of telephone interviews, can help many types of households by making it easier for them to complete the food stamp application or recertification process. Some state and local officials and community partners noted, however, that certain types of households may have difficulty using some methods. Moreover, some officials also described how technology and staffing challenges can hinder the use of these methods.

Advantages of Alternative Methods

According to federal and state officials we interviewed, alternative methods can help households in several ways, such as increasing flexibility, making it easier to receive case information or report changes to household circumstances, or increasing efficiency of application processing. In addition, community partner representatives from some states we reviewed said that the availability of telephone interviews helps reduce the stigma of applying for food stamp benefits caused by visiting an assistance office.

- *Increased flexibility.* Federal officials from the seven FNS regional offices said that alternative methods help households by reducing the number of visits a household makes to an assistance office or by providing additional ways to comply with program requirements. Moreover, all of the states in our survey that currently have on-line services and more than half of the states that currently operate call centers, reported that reducing the number of visits an individual must make to an office as a reason for implementing the alternative methods. For example, in Florida a household may submit an application or recertification through any one of the following access points -- on-line, mail, fax, community partner site, or in-person at the local assistance office. Additionally, in certain areas of Texas, it is possible for households to apply for food stamps without ever visiting a local assistance office because the state has made available phone interviews and on-line services. Reducing the number of required visits can be helpful for all households, according to state officials or community partner representatives in two of the states we reviewed.

- *Easier access to case information and ability to report changes.* According to officials in the five states we reviewed, alternative methods, such as call centers, automated voice response systems, or electronic case records, make it easier for households to access information about their benefits and report changes to household circumstances. For example, in Washington, a household may call the automated voice response system 24 hours a day, 7 days a week to immediately access case information, such as appointment times or whether their application has been received or is being processed. If the household has additional questions, they can call the call center where a call center agent can view their electronic case record and provide information on the status of their application, make decisions based on changes in household circumstances reported to them, inform them of what verification documents are needed or have been received, or perform other services.
- *Increased efficiency.* State or local officials from four of the states we reviewed said that implementation of document management/imaging systems improves application processing times, while local officials in two of the states said that call centers help caseworkers complete tasks more quickly. Furthermore, about half of the states in our survey that have call centers reported that increasing timeliness of application processing and reducing administrative costs were reasons for implementing them. State officials in Florida said that the document management/imaging system allows a caseworker to retrieve an electronic case record in seconds compared to retrieving paper case files that previously took up to 24 hours, allowing caseworkers to make eligibility decisions more quickly on a case. Additionally, a call center agent can process a change in household circumstances instantly while on the phone. Caseworkers in Pennsylvania said that implementation of a change reporting call center has reduced the number of calls to caseworkers at the local assistance office, which allows them to focus on interviewing households and processing applications more quickly. Officials from four states we reviewed also said that use of a document management/imaging system has resulted in fewer lost documents, which can reduce the burden on households of having to resubmit information.

According to some of the state officials and community partners we interviewed, the availability of alternative methods can be especially beneficial for working families or the elderly because it reduces barriers from transportation, child care or work responsibilities. For example, state officials in Florida explained that a working individual can complete a phone interview during their lunch break without taking time off of work to wait in line at the assistance office. In addition, state officials from three of the states we reviewed that have implemented CAP projects told us that they had experienced an increase in participation among SSI recipients and FNS and officials from two states said that households benefited from the simplified application process. In addition, state officials in Florida said that on-line services help elderly households that have designated representatives to complete the application on their behalf. For example, an elderly individual's adult child who is the appointed designated representative but lives out-of-state can apply and recertify for food stamp benefits for their parent without traveling to Florida.

However, some state and local officials and community partners we interviewed said certain types of households may have difficulty using certain alternative methods. For example, community partner representatives in two states that we reviewed said that those with limited English proficiency, elderly, immigrants, or those with mental disabilities may have difficulty using on-line applications. Local officials from Philadelphia said that the elderly and households with very low incomes may have trouble accessing computers to use on-line services and may not have someone helping them. A community partner in Florida told us that sometimes the elderly, illiterate, or those with limited English proficiency need a staff person to help them complete the on-line application. In addition, those with limited English proficiency, elderly, or those with mental disabilities may have difficulty navigating the call center phone system, according to officials from two states and community partners from another state that we reviewed. A community partner representative in Texas said that sometimes he calls the call center on behalf of the applicant because a household may have experienced difficulty or frustration in navigating the phone system.

Challenges to Using Alternative Methods

Although officials told us that alternative methods are helpful to many households, challenges from inadequate technology or staffing may limit the advantages of alternative methods. For example, state officials from Texas explained that on-line applications without electronic signature capability have limited benefit because households are still required to submit an actual signature through mail, fax, or in person after completing the on-line application. Texas state officials and community partner representatives told us that the lack of this capability limited its use and benefit to households. By contrast, Florida's application has electronic signature capability and Florida officials reported that, as of December 2006, about 93 percent of their applications are submitted on-line.

Call centers that do not have access to electronic records may not be as effective at answering callers' questions. Officials from Washington state and federal officials from an FNS regional office view the use of a document management/imaging system as a vital part of the call center system. Florida advocates said that households have received wrong information from call center agents and attribute the complaints in part to call center agents not having access to real-time electronic case records.

Florida recently expanded its document imaging system statewide, which they believe will help address these concerns.

Further, while four of the five states we reviewed implemented alternative methods in part to better manage increasing numbers of participants with reduced numbers of staff, the staffing challenges certain states experienced also limited the advantages of alternative methods. For example, inadequate numbers of staff or unskilled call center staff may reduce the level of service provided and limit the advantages to households of having a call center available to them. Texas and Florida have experienced significant staff reductions at a time of increased participation, which has affected implementation of alternative methods (see figs. 10 and 11).

In January 2006, Texas piloted in two counties a call center system run by a private contractor to assist state caseworkers in gathering the client information needed to determine households' eligibility for multiple programs, including food stamps. Initially, the contractor was responsible for a number of tasks such as scheduling interviews, assisting households with applications, gathering verification documents from households, and assembling electronic case records. A March 2006 FNS review of the system found several problems related to the performance of the contractor, such as inefficient application processing, long wait times and a high abandonment rate for individuals using the call center, and contractor call center agents providing incorrect or confusing information to callers. In May 2006, in response to a large backlog of food stamp applications and contractor performance problems, the state took back responsibility for processing food stamp applications, with the exception of receiving the applications, scanning documents, and scheduling interviews. In December 2006, Texas announced a plan to retain some functions originally envisioned to be performed by the private contractor and reduce the terms of the contract. In March 2007, Texas announced that it will terminate the contract with the existing private contractor and expects that all duties currently performed by the private contractor, such as operating the call centers, will conclude no later than November 2007. During the transition, some of the work will continue to be performed by subcontractors while Texas evaluates whether to hire state staff and develop systems for those tasks or use different contractors. Texas plans to assess whether they will continue to outsource some of the administrative support tasks, such as mailing notices and scanning documents.

Challenges

- State officials reported that between 2002 and 2006, through budget reductions the state reduced its eligibility staff by one-third while experiencing a 45 percent increase in the number of participants. The new system initially called for an additional reduction in staff and closure of about 100 local assistance offices. When implementation of the new system began, the state sent notices of impending layoffs to state eligibility staff and many of them left their positions as a result. In May 2006 when the state took back responsibility for processing applications, Texas announced that it would retain an additional 1,000 state workers and pay retention bonuses to keep state staff in place. The state also hired more than 900 temporary employees to help offices experiencing high turnover during the transition.
- Texas state officials told us that they underestimated the level of expertise and training the contractor's call center agents needed. For example, call center agents delayed the application process by sending applicants multiple requests for missing information, whereas a state caseworker would have known to use data-matching resources or other means to verify the information.
- In addition, state officials attributed Texas' recent increases in the payment and negative error rates to inexperienced staff handling a large increase in applications following Hurricanes Katrina and Rita.
- Texas also experienced technology challenges because the state's new automated case management system, which was developed several years before the legislative mandate to develop call centers, had to be retrofitted to work within the call center model. The private contractor offered an interim technical solution which was determined to be insufficient.

Source: GAO analysis.

Figure 10. Use of Alternative Access Methods in Texas.

Florida began its modernization initiative to save costs following state legislative direction. The initiative included closing about one-third of the local assistance offices and establishing community partnerships to serve as access locations. The state implemented alternative methods gradually by reinvesting funds saved from reducing staff and office leases into technology and training, and investing in community partnerships. The state strongly encourages households to apply on-line by directing individuals visiting the local assistance offices to computers and providing computers and training to community partners. State officials reported that as of December 2006, about 93 percent of applications were filed on-line. In addition, Florida created call centers that provide case and referral information and process reported changes.

Challenges

- State officials reported absorbing a 43 percent staff reduction at a time of increasing participation.
- The state has had difficulties providing adequate call center staff to handle the volume of calls. Due to long hold times, households have hung up and not received service, according to community partner representatives. State officials told us that they did not anticipate the large volume of callers when they designed the call center, but that they are working to address the problems.
- Community partner representatives and advocates told us that some community partners do not have the resources or training necessary to assist people with the food stamp application process.
- Florida's payment and negative error rates increased recently, and state officials attribute this in part to fewer staff handling a large increase in applications and disruption following Hurricane Wilma.

Source: GAO analysis.

Figure 11. Use of Alternative Access Methods in Florida.

While some states face challenges implementing alternative methods, Utah state officials said that they have successful call centers because they have implemented technology incrementally over time and because they use state caseworkers experienced in program rules. Utah state officials also reported having relatively low caseloads (180 per worker) compared with Texas (815 per worker, in 2005).

STATES REPORT TAKING ACTIONS TO MAINTAIN FOOD STAMP PROGRAM INTEGRITY WHILE USING ALTERNATIVE METHODS

To maintain program integrity while implementing alternative methods for applying and recertifying for food stamps, officials from the states we reviewed reported using a variety of strategies, some of which were in place long before implementation of the alternative access methods. Some states used finger imaging, electronic signatures, and special verification techniques to validate the identity of households using call centers or online services. In addition, states use databases to verify information provided by households and to follow up on discrepancies between information reported by the household and information obtained from other sources. Officials in the five states we reviewed did not believe that the use of alternative methods had increased fraud in the program. Further, despite concern that a lack of face-to-face interaction with caseworkers would lead to more households being denied benefits for procedural reasons, such as missing a scheduled interview, our limited analysis indicated no considerable fluctuations in the rate of procedural denials and officials from the states we reviewed reported taking actions to prevent them.

State Actions to Prevent Improper Food Stamp Payments and Fraud

Some states have taken several actions to prevent improper food stamp payments and fraud while implementing alternative methods. Nationally, states have systems in place to protect program integrity and the states we reviewed described how they prevent improper payments and fraud as they implement alternative access methods.

- *Finger imaging.* Nationwide, four states[17] currently use finger imaging of food stamp applicants to prevent households from applying more than once for benefits. FNS officials commented that the agency has not concluded that finger imaging enhances program integrity and that it may have a negative effect on program access by deterring certain households from applying.
- *Electronic signatures.* FNS reported in October 2006 that nine states use electronic signatures to validate the identity of on-line users of their systems. For example, Florida's on-line application asks applicants to click a button signifying that they are signing the application. Of the states we reviewed, Pennsylvania, Florida, and Washington have on-line services with electronic signatures.[18]
- *In-depth interview for high-risk cases.* In Florida, a case that is considered to have a greater potential for error or fraud is flagged as a "red track" case, and it receives an in-depth interview to more fully explore eligibility factors. FNS officials commented that Florida uses an abbreviated interview with most households and that their in-depth interview for red track cases may be equivalent to the standard interview process used in other states.
- *Special training for call center agents.* Call center agents in the five states we reviewed are trained to verify callers' identities by asking for specific personal information available in the file or in the states' records. Pennsylvania has developed specialized interview training, including a video, for eligibility workers on conducting telephone interviews of households applying or recertifying for the Food Stamp Program. One element of the training is how to detect misinformation being provided by a household. For example, if records indicate that a household member is currently incarcerated and benefits are being claimed for that person, call center agents are trained to probe for additional information. Similarly, Utah trains telephone interviewers to request more information if needed to clarify discrepancies in the case, such as a household reporting rent payments too high to be covered by the household's reported income.
- *Data matching.* States have used data matching systems for many years and all five states we reviewed used software either developed by the state or obtained through a third-party vendor to help with verification of household circumstances. For example, data matching software can match state food stamp caseloads against wage reporting

systems and other databases to identify unreported household income and assets. Utah and Washington have developed software that automatically compares information provided by applicants and recipients with information contained in state databases, such as income and employment information. State officials told us that using this software greatly reduces the burden on caseworkers, who would otherwise have to search multiple databases one at a time. In addition to requiring case workers to access state and federal data sources to verify information, Texas contracts with a private data vendor to obtain financial and other background information on food stamp applicants and recipients. After a household has started receiving benefits, states conduct additional data matching, and their systems generate a notice to the caseworker if there is a conflict between what the household reported and information obtained from another source. The information in these notices is investigated to ensure that recipients receive the proper level of benefits. Finally, about half of all states participate in the voluntary quarterly matching of their food stamp rolls with those of other states to detect individuals receiving food stamp benefits in more than one state at a time.

Food stamp officials in four of the states we reviewed said that they did not believe the use of alternative methods has increased the frequency of fraud and abuse in the program and officials in one state were unsure and collecting data to help determine whether the frequency of fraud had increased. Texas caseworkers, for example, told us they did not think telephone interviews increased fraud because they believed the verification conducted by caseworkers and the states' data matching system was sufficient. However, we have previously reported on the risk of improper payments and fraud in the food stamp program and since there is always risk of fraud and improper payments, particularly given the high volume of cases and the complexity of the program, it is important that states include additional controls when changing their processes and that states continually assess the adequacy of those controls for preventing fraud.

State Actions to Limit Procedural Denials

Some program experts have expressed concern that households would be denied for procedural reasons more frequently if they had less face-to-face interaction with caseworkers, although data have not borne out these concerns and states are taking actions to limit procedural denials. During our site visits, some officials reported examples of procedural denials resulting from alternative methods. For example, community group representatives in Florida said that some households were denied benefits because they could not get through to a call center agent to provide required verification in time. However, they also acknowledged that procedural denials due to not providing verification were frequent prior to the state implementing these methods. In addition, Texas officials said that some households were denied benefits for missing scheduled interviews when the private contractor was late in mailing notices of the interview appointments.

Our limited analysis of FNS data for the five states we reviewed found no considerable fluctuations in the rate of procedural denials between fiscal years 2000 and 2005. However, a household's failure to provide verification documents was the most common procedural reason for denial, suspension, or termination of benefits in the five states we reviewed. States we visited described their efforts to help households use alternative methods and prevent procedural denials for households that are not seen in person by case workers. Examples of actions the states we reviewed took to prevent procedural denials include: reviewing actions taken for cases that are denied, training caseworkers on preventing improper denials, routinely correcting addresses from returned mail, and developing automated system changes to prevent caseworkers from prematurely denying a case. For example, Utah trains its caseworkers to inform households of all deadlines, and their application tracking software automatically generates a list of households that have not scheduled an interview. This list is used by caseworkers to send notices to the households. Washington uses its document imaging center staff to process case actions associated with returned mail, including quickly correcting addresses.

CONCLUSIONS

Over the last several years and for a variety of reasons, many states have changed their food stamp certification and recertification processes to enable households to make fewer visits to the local assistance office. Given our findings, it is important for states to consider the needs of all types of households when developing alternative ways of accessing food stamp benefits. Despite making major changes in their systems, FNS and the states have little information on the effects of the alternative methods on the Food Stamp Program, including what factors contribute to successful implementation, whether these methods are improving access to benefits for target groups, and how best to ensure program integrity. Without up-to-date information about what methods states are using and the factors that contribute to successful implementation of alternative methods, states and the federal government most likely will continue to invest in large-scale changes to their certification and recertification processes without knowing what works and in what contexts. Although FNS is beginning to study state efforts in this regard, these studies are not designed to systematically evaluate whether specific methods contributed to achieving positive outcomes. In addition, FNS has not thoroughly analyzed the data received from states implementing waivers of the face- to-face interview to determine, for example, whether it should allow states to use telephone interviews in lieu of face-to-face interviews for all types of households without a waiver. Further, while FNS is using its Website to disseminate information about promising practices, the information available is not up-to-date, making it difficult to easily locate current information about specific practices. Enhancing the research, collection and dissemination of promising practices could be an important resource for states that want to provide households effective alternatives to visiting local assistance offices to receive food stamp benefits.

RECOMMENDATIONS FOR EXECUTIVE ACTION

To improve USDA's ability to assess the effectiveness of its funded efforts, we recommend that the Secretary of Agriculture take the following actions:

- direct FNS and the Economic Research Service to work together to enhance their research agendas to include projects that would complement ongoing research efforts and determine the effect of alternative methods on program access, decision accuracy, and administrative costs. Such projects would reliably identify the alternative methods that are effective and the factors that contribute to their success; and

- direct FNS to conduct analyses of data received from states implementing waivers or demonstration projects waiving the face-to- face interview and require states implementing waivers or demonstration projects to collect and report data that would facilitate such analyses. Such analyses would identify the effect of the waivers on outcomes such as payment accuracy and could help determine whether the use of the waiver should be further expanded or inform whether regulations should be changed to allow telephone interviews for all households without documenting hardship.

In addition, we recommend that the Secretary of Agriculture help states implement alternative methods to provide access to the Food Stamp Program by directing FNS to disseminate and regularly update information on practices states are using to implement alternative access methods to the traditional application and recertification process. The information would not be merely a listing of practices attempted, but would include details on what factors or contexts seemed to make a particular practice successful and what factors may have reduced its effectiveness.

Agency Comments

We provided a draft of this report to the U.S. Department of Agriculture for review and comment. We met with FNS and ERS officials on April 16, 2007, to obtain their comments. In general, the officials agreed with our findings, conclusions, and recommendations. They discussed the complexity and variability of state modernization efforts and the related challenges of researching the effects of these efforts. For example, policy changes, organizational restructuring, and the engagement of community organizations in the application process may occur simultaneously with implementation of alternative methods and play a significant role in state and client experiences. Having multiple interrelated factors creates challenges for researching the effects of modernization efforts. Nonetheless, the officials highlighted steps the agency is taking to monitor and evaluate state implementation of alternative access methods. First, the officials commented that as modernization evolves, FNS is using its administrative reporting system to consistently and routinely track changes in state program performance in the areas of application timeliness, food stamp participation by subgroups, payment accuracy, and administrative costs. Second, they stated that the two related FNS-funded studies currently underway will be comparing performance data from the case study states with data from similar states; however, this analysis will not determine whether certain modernization efforts caused changes in performance. Third, they stated that FNS plans to analyze data they are collecting from states as part of the administrative waiver process to determine the effect of telephone interviews on payment accuracy. Finally, ERS officials noted that Food Stamp Program access is an area in which the agency continues to solicit research from the private sector as well as other government agencies and that ERS makes data available to support these research efforts. FNS and ERS also provided us with technical comments, which we incorporated where appropriate.

We are sending copies of this report to the Secretary of Agriculture, appropriate congressional committees, and other interested parties. We will also make copies available to others upon request.

In addition, the report will be available at no charge on GAO's Web site at http://www.gao.gov.

If you or your staff have any questions about this report, please contact me at (202) 512-7215 or nilsens@gao.gov. Contact points for our Offices of Congressional Relations and Public Affairs may be found on the last page of this report. GAO staff who made major contributions to this report are listed in appendix III.

Sincerely,

Sigurd R. Nilsen,
Director Education, Workforce, and
Income Security Issues

APPENDIX I: OBJECTIVES, SCOPE, AND METHODOLOGY

To understand what alternatives states are using to improve program access and what is known about the results of using these methods, we examined: (1) what alternative methods to the traditional application and recertification process are states using to increase program access; (2) what is known about the results of these methods, particularly on program access for target groups, decision accuracy, and administrative costs; and (3) what actions have states taken to maintain program integrity while implementing alternative methods.

To address these issues, we surveyed food stamp administrators in the 50 states and the District of Columbia, conducted four state site visits (Florida, Texas, Utah, and Washington) and one set of semi-structured telephone interviews (Pennsylvania), analyzed data provided by the Food and Nutrition Service (FNS) and the selected states, reviewed relevant studies, and held discussions with program stakeholders, including officials at FNS headquarters and regional offices, and representatives of advocacy organizations. We performed our work from September 2006 to March 2007 in accordance with generally accepted government auditing standards.

Survey of State Food Stamp Administrators

To learn about state-level use of alternative methods to help households access the Food Stamp Program, we conducted a Web-based survey of food stamp administrators in the 50 states and the District of Columbia. The survey was conducted between December 2006 and February 2007 with 100 percent of state food stamp administrators responding. The survey included questions about the use of alternative methods to provide access to the program, including mail-in procedures, call centers, on-line services, and other technologies that support program access. In addition, we asked about the reasons for implementing these methods, whether states had conducted evaluations of the methods, what measures states used to evaluate the performance of the methods, and additional assistance needed from FNS.

Because this was not a sample survey, there are no sampling errors. However, the practical difficulties of conducting any survey may introduce nonsampling errors, such as variations in how respondents interpret questions and their willingness to offer accurate responses. We took steps to minimize nonsampling errors, including pre-testing draft instruments and using a Web-based administration system. Specifically, during survey development, we pre-tested draft instruments with officials in Washington, Arizona, Utah, and Wisconsin in October and November 2006. In the pretests, we were generally interested in the clarity of the questions and the flow and layout of the survey. For example, we wanted to ensure definitions used in the surveys were clear and known to the respondents, categories provided in closed-ended questions were complete and exclusive, and the ordering of survey sections and the questions within each section was appropriate. We also used in-depth interviewing techniques to evaluate the answers of pretest participants, and interviewers judged that all the respondents' answers to the questions were based on reliable information.

On the basis of the pre-tests, the Web instrument underwent some slight revisions. A second step we took to minimize nonsampling errors was using a Web-based survey. By allowing respondents to enter their responses directly into an electronic instrument, this method automatically created a record for each respondent in a data file and eliminated the need for and the errors (and costs) associated with a manual data entry process. To further minimize errors, programs used to analyze the survey data were independently verified to ensure the accuracy of this work.

After the survey was closed, we made comparisons between select items from our survey data and other national-level data.[19] We found our survey data were reasonably consistent with the other data set. On the basis of our comparisons, we believe our survey data are sufficient for the purposes of our work.

State Site Visits and Structured Interviews

We conducted four site visits (Florida, Texas, Utah, and Washington) and one set of semi-structured telephone interviews (Pennsylvania). We selected states that have at least one FNS-approved waiver of the face-to- face interview requirement and reflect some variation in state participation rates. We also considered recommendations from FNS officials, advocacy group representatives, or researchers. We made in- depth reviews for each state we selected. We interviewed state officials administering and developing policy for the Food Stamp Program, local officials in the assistance offices and call centers where services are provided, and representatives from community-based organizations that provide food assistance.

Reviews of FNS Data and Relevant Studies

To supplement the information gathered through our site visits and in- depth reviews, we analyzed data provided by FNS for the states we reviewed. These analyses allowed us to include state trends for specific measures (Program Access Index, monthly participation, payment accuracy, administrative costs, and reasons for benefit denials) in our interviews with officials. To review the reasons for benefit denials, we used FNS's quality control (QC) system data of negative cases used in error rate calculations. Specifically, we looked at the number and percentage of cases denied, terminated, or suspended by the recorded reason for the action in the five states we reviewed for fiscal years 2000 through 2005. Though our data allowed us to examine patterns in these areas before and after a method was implemented, we did not intend to make any statements about the effectiveness of methods implemented in the states we visited and reviewed. Instead, we were interested in gaining some insight through our interviews on how alternative methods may have affected state trends. Based on discussions with and documentation obtained from FNS officials, and interviews with FNS staff during site visits, we determined that these data are sufficiently reliable for our limited review of state trends.

In addition, we selected and reviewed several studies and reports that relate to the use of alternative methods to increase food stamp program access. These studies included food stamp participation outcome evaluations that were funded by FNS and the Economic Research Service (ERS) and focused on practices aimed to improve access to the Food Stamp Program. To identify the selected studies, we conducted library and Internet searches for research published on food stamp program access since 1990, interviewed agency officials to identify completed and ongoing studies on program access, and reviewed bibliographies that focused on program access concerns. For each selected study, we determined whether the study's findings were generally reliable. Two GAO social science analysts evaluated the methodological soundness of the studies, and the validity of the results and conclusions that were drawn.

The studies we selected and reviewed include:

- U.S. Department of Agriculture, Economic Research Service, *Food Stamp Program Access Study: Final Report,* by Bartlett, S., N. Burstein, and W. Hamilton, Abt Associates Inc. (Washington, D.C.: November 2004).
- U.S. Department of Agriculture, Economic Research Service, *Evaluation of the USDA Elderly Nutrition Demonstrations,* by Cody, S. and J. Ohls, Mathematica Policy Research, Inc. (Washington, D.C.: May 2005).
- U.S. Department of Agriculture, Food and Nutrition Services, Office of Analysis, Nutrition and Evaluation, *Evaluation of Food Stamp Research Grants to Improve Access Through New Technology and Partnerships*, by Sheila Zedlewski, David Wittenburg, Carolyn O'Brien, Robin Koralek, Sandra Nelson, and Gretchen Rowe. (Alexandria, Va.: September 2005).
- U.S. Department of Agriculture, Food and Consumer Service, *Evaluation of SSI/FSP Joint Processing Alternatives Demonstration*, by Carol Boussy, Russell H. Jackson, and Nancy Wemmerus. (Alexandria, Va: January 2000.
- Combined Application Project Evaluations submitted to FNS by seven states: Florida, Massachusetts, Mississippi, North Carolina, South Carolina, Texas, and Washington.

Appendix II: State-by-State Use of Alternative Methods and Waivers of the Face-to-Face Interview

	Mail-in Procedures								
State	Submit application	Report changes	Submit recertification	On-line services	Call centers	Face-to-face waiver at application	Face-to-face waiver at recertification	CAP	Elderly demonstration project
Alabama	•	•	•						
Alaska	•	•	•						
Arizona	•	•	•	•	•				
Arkansas	•	•	•				√		
California	•	•	•				√		
Colorado	•	•	•						
Connecticut	•	•	•	♦			√		
Delaware	•	•	•	•			√		
District of Columbia	•	•			•				
Florida	•	•	•	•	•	√	√	√	√
Georgia	•	•		♦	•				
Hawaii	•	•	•						
Idaho	•	•	•	•	•				
Illinois	•	•	•	♦	•		√		
Indiana	•	•	•	♦	♦	√	√		
Iowa	•	•	•	♦	•				
Kansas	•	•	•	•	♦				
Kentucky	•	•		♦				▲	
Louisiana	•	•	•				√	▲	
Maine	•	•	•						
Maryland	•	•	•	•	•				
Massachusetts	•	•	•	•	♦		√	√	
Michigan	•	•	•						
Minnesota	•	•	•						
Mississippi	•	•	•	♦				√	
Missouri	•	•	•						
Montana	•	•	•						
Nebraska	•	•	•						

(Continued).

	Mail-in Procedures								
State	Submit application	Report changes	Submit recertification	On-line services	Call centers	Face-to-face waiver at application	Face-to-face waiver at recertification	CAP	Elderly demonstration project
Nevada	●	●	●		●				
New Hampshire	●	●	●	♦	●				
New Jersey	●			●				▲	
New Mexico	●	●	●				√		
New York	●	●	●	♦	●		√	√	
North Carolina	●	●	●				√	√	
North Dakota	●	●	●						
Ohio	●	●	●		●		√		
Oklahoma	●	●	●		♦				
Oregon	●	●	●						
Pennsylvania	●	●	●	●	●		√	√	
Rhode Island	●	●	●	♦					
South Carolina	●	●	●				√	√	√
South Dakota	●	●	●				√		
Tennessee	●	●	●	♦	●		√		
Texas	●	●	●	●	●		√	√	
Utah	●	●	●	♦	●	√	√		
Vermont	●	●	●						
Virginia	●	●	●	●	●				
Washington	●	●	●	●	●		√	√	
West Virginia	●	●	●	●	●				
Wisconsin	●	●		●					
Wyoming	●	●	●						
Total	51	50	46	26	23	3	20	13	2

√ State has implemented project or waiver

▲ Project approved, not yet implemented

● Services available to households within the state

♦ State has begun development of a call center or on-line services

Source: GAO survey and FNS.

RELATED GAO PRODUCTS

Food Stamp Program: FNS Could Improve Guidance and Monitoring to Help Ensure Appropriate Use of Noncash Categorical Eligibility. GAO-07-465. Washington, D.C.: March 28, 2007.

Food Stamp Program: Payment Errors and Trafficking Have Declined despite Increased Program Participation. GAO-07-422T. January 31, 2007.

Food Stamp Trafficking: FNS Could Enhance Program Integrity by Better Targeting Stores Likely to Traffic and Increasing Penalties. GAO-07-53. Washington, D.C.: October 13, 2006.

Improper Payments: Federal and State Coordination Needed to Report National Improper Payment Estimates on Federal Programs. GAO-06-347. Washington, D.C.: April 14, 2006.

Food Stamp Program: States Have Made Progress Reducing Payment Errors, and Further Challenges Remain. GAO-05-245. Washington, D.C.: May 5, 2005.

Food Stamp Program: Farm Bill Options Ease Administrative Burden, but Opportunities Exist to Streamline Participant Reporting Rules among Programs. GAO-04-916. Washington, D.C.: September 16, 2004.

Food Stamp Program: Steps Have Been Taken to Increase Participation of Working Families, but Better Tracking of Efforts Is Needed. GAO-04-346. Washington, D.C.: March 5, 2004.

Financial Management: Coordinated Approach Needed to Address the Government's Improper Payments Problems. GAO-02-749. Washington, D.C.: August 9, 2002.

Food Stamp Program: States' Use of Options and Waivers to Improve Program Administration and Promote Access. GAO-02-409. Washington, D.C.: February 22, 2002.

Executive Guide: Strategies to Manage Improper Payments: Learning from Public and Private Sector Organizations. GAO-02-69G. Washington, D.C.: October 2001.

Food Stamp Program: States Seek to Reduce Payment Errors and Program Complexity. GAO-01-272. Washington D.C.: January 19, 2001.

Food Stamp Program: Better Use of Electronic Data Could Result in Disqualifying More Recipients Who Traffic Benefits. GAO/RCED-00-61. Washington D.C.: March 7, 2000.

Food Assistance: Reducing the Trafficking of Food Stamp Benefits. GAO/T-RCED-00-250. Washington D.C.: July 19, 2000.

Food Stamp Program: Information on Trafficking Food Stamp Benefits. GAO/RCED-98-77. Washington D.C.: March 26, 1998.

REFERENCES

[1] Preliminary FNS data indicate that participation continued to grow to nearly 27 million people receiving about $30 billion in food stamp benefits in fiscal year 2006.

[2] In this report, we refer to all 50 states and the District of Columbia as states.

[3] Reimbursements for food stamp administrative costs in 44 states are adjusted each year to subtract certain food stamp administrative costs that have already been factored into these states' Temporary Assistance for Needy Families (TANF) grants. As a result, these

states receive less than 50 percent of their administrative costs. See GAO, *Food Stamp Program: States Face Reduced Federal Reimbursement for Administrative Costs,* GAO/RCED/AIMD-99-231 (Washington D.C.: July 23, 1999).

[4] As GAO and others have reported previously, following the passage of PRWORA, there is evidence that food stamp participation dropped as eligible recipients did not apply for food stamps because they incorrectly assumed that if they were ineligible for TANF, they were also ineligible for food stamps. See U.S. GAO, *Food Stamp Program: Various Factors Have Led to Declining Participation,* GAO/RCED-99-185 (Washington D.C.: July 1999) for more details.

[5] The Farm Security and Rural Investment Act of 2002 (the 2002 Farm Bill) included provisions intended to simplify program administration, such as allowing states the option of using simplified/semiannual reporting systems for most households, not just those with earned income. FNS reported in October 2006 that 47 states have adopted some form of simplified reporting, allowing most households to report changes only when their income rises above 130 percent of the poverty level. A FNS study suggested that simplified reporting policies have contributed to a reduction in the food stamp payment error rate.

[6] For more information on food stamp payment accuracy and trafficking, see Food Stamp Program: States Have Made Progress Reducing Payment Errors, and Further Challenges Remain, GAO-05-245. (Washington, D.C.: May 5, 2005) and Food Stamp Trafficking: FNS Could Enhance Program Integrity by Better Targeting Stores Likely to Traffic and Increasing Penalties, GAO-07-53. (Washington, D.C.: Oct. 13, 2006).

[7] See appendix II for state-by-state information on use of alternative methods.

[8] Utah began piloting an on-line application with electronic signature capability in March 2007. Because this was after the time our survey was conducted, Utah is not included in the 14 states that currently provide on-line services. FNS reported in October 2006 that nine states nationwide allow applicants to submit the application with an electronic signature.

[9] See appendix II for names of states with administrative waivers that allow substitution of a telephone interview for the face-to-face interview.

[10] Utah began piloting an on-line application with electronic signature capability in March 2007. Because this was after the time our survey was conducted, Utah is not included in the 14 states that currently provide on-line services.

[11] *Evaluation of the USDA Elderly Nutrition Demonstrations*, Scott Cody and James Ohls, Mathematica Policy Research, Inc., May 2005.

[12] In addition to studies that are under way, the fiscal year 2008 Food Nutrition and Consumer Services budget request, which includes FNS, includes $2 million to support Food Stamp Modernization and Innovation Projects to study the impact of new Food Stamp Program service delivery models on program access, payment accuracy, and administrative costs.

[13] State Best Practices Improving Food Stamp Program Access, USDA, FNS, (June 2002).

[14] Advocacy groups such as the American Public Human Services Association and the Food Research Action Center also make information available on food stamp outreach and access in best practices guides, on their Web sites, or through conferences.

[15] Food Stamp Program: Steps Have Been Taken to Increase Participation of Working Families, but Better Tracking of Efforts Is Needed, GAO-04-346 (Washington, D.C.: March 5, 2004).

[16] Combined Application Projects (CAP) allow one-person SSI households to file a shortened food stamp application form and waive the face-to-face interview requirement.

[17] Texas, California, New York, and Arizona.

[18] Utah also began piloting an on-line application with electronic signature capability in March 2007.

[19] We compared our Web-based survey data to data reported by FNS in the *2006 State Options Report.*

In: Hunger in America: Issues and Assistance
Editor: Gaston T. LaBue, pp. 119-124
ISBN: 978-1-60692-803-5

Chapter 5

TESTIMONY FOR THE COMMITTEE ON AGRICULTURE'S SUB-COMMITTEE ON DEPARTMENT OPERATIONS, OVERSIGHT, NUTRITION AND FORESTRY, ON THE SHORT AND LONG TERM EFFECTS OF HUNGER IN AMERICA

George Manalo-LeClair

July 23, 2008

Good Morning, Mr. Chair and Members of the Committee.

My name is George Manalo-LeClair and I am Senior Legislative Director for California Food Policy Advocates. CFPA is a statewide public policy and advocacy organization whose mission is to improve access to nutritious and affordable food for low-income Californians.

I appreciate the opportunity to testify today, as California has much to offer to this committee's consideration of the short and long term effects of hunger in America.

First, we have undertaken the largest statewide health survey in the country and found the problem of food insecurity is enormous in scope and impact.

Second, as our state has sought to address the problem, policymakers have acknowledged and quantified the contribution that Food Stamp Program benefits make, not only to families, but also to our state and local economies.

Third, building upon this economic benefit, I'd like to make a request for swift action to provide California residents immediate relief in these tough times.

Food Insecurity in California

Let's start with the problem of food insecurity in California. Though California has been number one in food and agriculture production in the U.S. for more than fifty years, we have millions of people struggling to put food on the table. We know this because in 2001, and biennially since, the University of California has conducted a large scale, statewide study, called the California Health Interview Survey (CHIS), to assess a broad range of health conditions, including food insecurity.

CHIS has been a massive and reliable effort. CHIS is the largest state health survey and one of the largest health surveys in the country. Because of its large sample size, with over 50,000 households interviewed, it generates statistically significant findings for the entire state and for most of our 58 counties. This biennial survey is conducted by the University of California at Los Angeles in collaboration with the California Department of Public Health, the Department of Health Care Services and the Public Health Institute.

UCLA publishes the food insecurity findings every two years. I have been a co□author of this research since its inception and have participated in each biennial release.

At first, the scope of the food□insecurity problem seemed unbelievably large, but over time the results have painted a consistent picture. According to the most recent CHIS release in 2007, approximately 2.5 million low□income adults in California struggle to put food on the table[1]. But this figure doesn't capture the full extent of the problem since this survey measures food insecurity only among adults. We know that these adults are not alone in their struggles, and we know that despite their best efforts, parents aren't always able to shield their kids from the consequences of hunger and food insecurity. Before I quantify the full dimension of this comprehensive understanding of how food insecurity affects real households, let me give you an example of one parent's attempt to protect her children.

Several years ago I met a woman who was in a culinary training program in our state's prosperous Silicon Valley. Money was really tight for her and despite working around food all day, she just did not have enough to provide for her family. At the dinner table she'd be hungry, but there wasn't always enough food for her children and for her. So to keep herself from taking food from her children, she'd pour herself a big glass of water. And then another. And sometimes another so that she would fool herself into feeling full and not be tempted to take food that would otherwise go to the children.

Not all parents are this successful in shielding their children. Based on the CHIS data, more than 7.5 million other people living with these adults also experience food insecurity. Given that these households share dinner tables, in many cases they must also share in their struggles with food. Understood this way, over 9 million people in California – perhaps a quarter of the population – are being affected by these struggles[2].

The wealth of data provided by the CHIS survey presents a surprising snapshot of who is hungry in the state:

- In California, hard work is no guarantee against hunger; the majority of households experiencing food insecurity are employed. Low wages and high rents mean many working families don't always have enough resources for food.

- In California, hunger does not discriminate. Food insecurity affects people of many races, though Latinos and African□Americans experience it at higher rates. Immigrants are among the hardest hit.
- Food insecurity in California also knows no boundaries as it is prevalent in all 58 counties. But some communities are hit much harder than others. It is ironic that the counties with the greatest agricultural production also have the greatest percentage of their population struggling with food.

Families with children are much more likely than families without children to struggle to put food on the table in California.

Consequences of Food Insecurity in California

It is clear that those lacking consistent access to adequate food suffer profound consequences. Other panelists today are going to go into greater detail on the health, employment and academic consequences of food insecurity. I'd also like to acknowledge the connections we have seen and measured, most notably that children in very low food□insecure households miss more school and do less well academically. And that those adults with food insecurity who experience health problems, such as diabetes and other obesity related conditions, have significantly more complications, more hospitalizations and more trips to the emergency room because of their food insecurity. One challenging finding is that in California those experiencing food insecurity are more likely to be overweight or obese. The remarkably steep price tag of obesity to our state – and the nation □□ is well documented.[3]

Addressing the Problem

The common factor among all of these struggling Californians is a lack of income. Policy action to increase wages, to make housing more affordable, and to adequately provide supports for the working poor like child care and health care would go a very long way to address the problem.

Short of this, we need a strong nutrition safety net. However, the CHIS data make it clear that current efforts are failing to make much progress in providing food security for low□income Californians.

Problems with Food Stamps in California

One of the most troubling findings of the California Health Interview Survey was the severe underutilization of the Food Stamp Program. More than 77 percent of those households identified as experiencing food insecurity in California who had qualifying incomes were not participating in the program. This means that essential help – that Congress put in place precisely for these people in this predicament -- is not getting to those most in need.

These CHIS findings are consistent with USDA research on food stamp participation in California. California has one of the worst food stamp participation rates in the country, and USDA estimates that over 2 million eligible Californians are not receiving food stamps[4]. If more Californians were receiving these valuable nutrition benefits, the problem of food insecurity discussed earlier would be greatly reduced.

The average monthly benefit per person in California is now just over $100. With rising food costs, this amount falls short of providing families with an adequate diet, but it certainly could make a tremendous difference for those not currently participating. Unfortunately, a number of state and federal rules make it difficult for struggling households, especially working families, even to participate. More than 70 percent of the households eligible for food stamps in California are working households.[5] According to USDA, California has the worst rate of food stamp participation among working people in the country. Just 35 percent of eligible working households in California participate in food stamps.[6]

When struggling working families don't get food stamps, it is not just the families that miss out but our economy as well. As CFPA's report *Lost Dollars, Empty Plates* points out, poor participation hurts our economy as well. California is passing up over $2 billion a year in federal nutrition benefits. This money would certainly help families, but in addition it could generate close to $4 billion annually in economic activity.

Capturing the Economic Benefits of Food Stamps to California

Policymakers in California are working to improve the reach of food stamps in our state. In response to interest from state legislators, the non-partisan Legislative Analyst's Office published a policy brief that has helped capture the economic benefits of food stamps to the state.[7]

The direct benefits of food stamps to families in our state are clear. But our analyst discovered that food stamps can also have economic benefits for our state and local economies. Under this analysis, food stamp dollars can lead to increased spending on taxable items. Though food is not taxed in our state and food stamp law prohibits taxes on food stamp purchases, increased food stamp funding nonetheless can actually increase state general fund revenues. This is so because when families get food stamps there is indeed increased spending on food but, in addition, resources are freed up in tight family budgets to be spent on taxable items such as clothes and shoes. Under this so-called "premise," this food stamp infusion generates about 45% of the value of the food stamps in taxable activity. With a state share of the sales tax pegged at 5%, one can see that increased food stamp spending can have a significant and positive impact on our state's strained general fund. And, because local communities receive a share of sales tax revenues (and in many cases add on to the sales tax), there are significant benefits from increased food stamp participation for local jurisdictions as well.

While this analysis falls short of the standard of peer-reviewed research, it is nonetheless embraced by the legislature, the Schwarzenegger Administration and advocates. Recognizing this, this analysis deserves further considerations and the Food Stamp Program deserves further investment. If Food Stamp Program participation were maximized in California, our state and counties could realize over $70 million a year in increased revenues. Given our state's fiscal crisis, we can use all the help we can get.

Taking Action

Recent Progress

Some help is already on the way, thanks to changes in the recently passed Farm Bill. We want to thank the Chair and members for your efforts to improve food stamps. The actions taken will help stop the erosion of food stamp benefits, will provide additional relief for working families with high child care costs, and help remove several disincentives to savings and asset development.

California stands to be a big winner with these changes. Support for nutrition will increase by an estimated $700 million dollars over the next five years. More than 800,000 California residents will feel these benefits.

While we are very grateful for this new investment, given the scope of the problem we are compelled to ask for additional action. We need to bring benefits to those struggling families who aren't participating in food stamps and we need to improve benefits for those that are. California needs a combination of actions which:

1. Simplify the program and improve access for working people who often can't complete program requirements because of work commitments.
2. Increase benefits not only to address rising food costs and to better support a healthy diet but also to better offset the 'costs' of participating in food stamps (long waits, lots of paperwork, many trips to the food stamp office) to families.
3. Extend aid to populations whose participation in food stamps is currently limited, such as legal immigrants and childless adults.

Congressional proposals already exist which would continue the progress already made by the Farm Bill and help families meet the demands of rising food prices. There are a number of provisions from the Chair's "*Nourish Act*" that were not incorporated in the Farm Bill that would help – most notably a restoration of benefits to legal immigrants who are currently denied help. The McGovern□Emerson "*Feeding America's Families Act*" has additional provisions, which if enacted would further improve benefits, help vulnerable childless adults, and further support savings and asset development. If Congress were to enact the provisions found in these two pieces of legislation, the pain of hunger would be lessened in our state.

A New Opportunity to Help Struggling Families and Our Economy

We will soon have an updated picture of the problem of food insecurity, as a new round of health survey data has been collected for the next CHIS report. Though updated, it still won't capture the most recent impacts of rising food and gas prices and other struggles. Our state legislature recently convened hearings on the topic and it was clear things were getting worse for low income residents: Average gas prices over $4.51 a gallon. Double digit increases for basic foods like bread and eggs. There have been increased demands for emergency food and food stamps. More needs to be done.

Our state economy needs help, too. We have an enormous budget shortfall – currently estimated at more than $15 billion. Unemployment is rising with preliminary estimates for June of a 6.9% unemployment rate. And we have been hit hard by the mortgage and lending crisis.

A short-term boost in food stamp benefits could help our struggling families and our struggling economy. The annual adjustment in food stamp benefits scheduled for October 1st will fall well short of providing what struggling families need for a bare- bones diet. Because the data used to calculate these benefit levels is already out of date, the new increase – on the day it is delivered --may already be more than $40 a month less than what a family of four needs to purchase a minimally adequate diet. Given this forecast, swift action is needed.

We are pleased to hear that Speaker Pelosi is considering including food stamps in an economic recovery package. We strongly support efforts to provide a temporary boost in basic food stamp benefit levels to help people afford a basic healthy diet. We would welcome the opportunity to help the Committee shape such a package -- its passage would minimize hunger by giving families a boost to meet these rising demands.

We also need this boost to help our state's struggling economy.

Given the importance of agriculture and the food industry to our state's economy, such action would go a long way in improving our fiscal situation. We hope that any new stimulus package would include this much-needed economic spark.

Thank you for your consideration

References

[1] UCLA Food Insecurity Brief, June 2007. http://www.healthpolicy.ucla.edu/pubs/publication.asp?pubID=225

[2] Shared Tables, Shared Struggles. CFPA. November 2007. http://www.cfpa.net/press/shared 2007/shared tables shared struggles 2007.pdf

[3] The Economic Costs Of Physical Inactivity, Obesity, And Overweight In California Adults, State Department of Health Care Services http://www.wellness taskforce.org/PDF/obese.pdf

[4] Reaching those in need. USDA. October 2007. http://www.fns.usda.gov/OANE/MENU/Published/FSP/FILES/Participation/Reaching 2005.pdf

[5] Comparison of Participation Rates Working vs. Non Working. CFPA. April 2001. http://www.cfpa.net/foodstamps/Participation/workpart.pdf

[6] State Participation Rates for the Working Poor. USDA. http://www.fns.usda.gov/OANE/MENU/Published/FSP/FILES/Participation/WorkingPoor2003.pdf

[7] LAO Budget Analysis Food Stamp Program. http://www.lao.ca.gov/analysis2004/healthss/hss20foodstampsanl04.htm

In: Hunger in America: Issues and Assistance
Editor: Gaston T. LaBue, pp. 125-131
ISBN: 978-1-60692-803-5

Chapter 6

STATEMENT OF DR. MARK NORD, SOCIOLOGIST, BEFORE THE AGRICULTURE SUBCOMMITTEE ON DEPARTMENT OPERATIONS, OVERSIGHT, NUTRITION, AND FORESTRY, JULY 23, 2008, HEARING ON THE SHORT AND LONG TERM IMPACTS OF HUNGER

Mr. Chairman and Members of the Committee, my name is Mark Nord, and I am a sociologist with the USDA's Economic Research Service. My main area of expertise is measuring and monitoring household food security—the extent to which households can consistently afford adequate food. I appreciate the opportunity to speak to you today about how USDA measures household food security and to provide an overview of recent food security statistics. I am accompanied by a representative of USDA's Food and Nutrition Service, who will also be available to answer questions.

Food security is a foundation for a healthy and well-nourished population—and food security statistics are a measure of the strength of that foundation. Information on unmet food need is of particular interest to USDA because of its responsibility for the Federal food and nutrition assistance programs.

I will begin with two or three salient food security statistics and then go behind those statistics to describe how households' food security was measured. Understanding the specific food conditions households reported in order to be classified as food insecure, or as having very low food security, may provide policy officials the best sense of what the food security numbers mean and how serious the conditions described by the statistics are. I will then conclude with a few further national-level statistics.

HOUSEHOLD FOOD SECURITY IN THE UNITED STATES, 2006

Most Americans can afford to put enough healthful food on the table each day. USDA estimates that slightly more than 89 percent of U.S. households were *food secure* throughout the entire year in 2006 (figure 1). Food secure households had access at all times to enough food for an active, healthy life for all household members. The remaining 12.6 million households (10.9 percent) were food insecure at some time during the year.

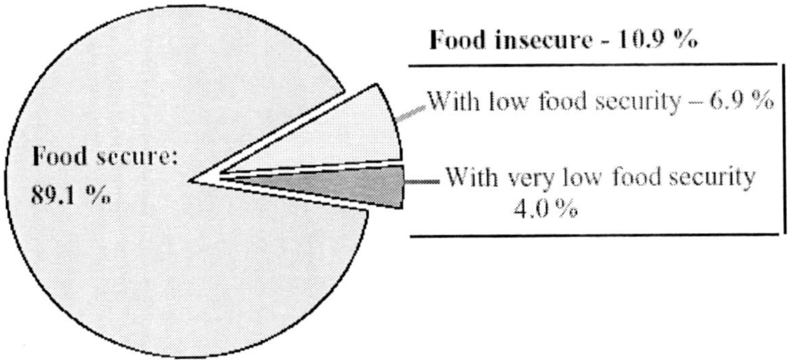

Source: Calculated by USDA, Economic Research Service using data from the December 2006 Current Population Survey Food Security Supplement.

Figure 1. Food Security of U.S. households, 2006.

About two-thirds of food-insecure households—those with *low food security*—obtained enough food to avoid substantial disruptions in eating patterns and food intake, using a variety of coping strategies such as eating less varied diets, participating in Federal food and nutrition assistance programs, or obtaining emergency food from community food pantries or emergency kitchens. But 4.6 million households (4.0 percent of all U.S. households) had *very low food security*—that is, they were food insecure to the extent that eating patterns of one or more household members were disrupted and their food intake reduced, at least some time during the year, because they couldn't afford enough food.

Behind the Statistics: How Does USDA Measure Household Food Security?

USDA monitors the food security of the Nation's households through an annual food security survey conducted by the U.S. Census Bureau. The survey is administered each December as a supplement to the Current Population Survey (CPS)—the same survey that provides monthly employment and unemployment statistics and annual income and poverty statistics. A nationally representative sample of about 45,000 households complete the food security survey each year.

The food security of each interviewed household is assessed by a series of questions about behaviors, conditions, and experiences that are related to households' food access. The questions cover a wide range of severity of food access problems, from worrying that food will run out to not eating for a whole day. Each question asks whether the condition or behavior occurred at any time during the previous 12 months and specifies a lack of money as the reason for the behavior or condition in question so that reduced food intake due to voluntary fasting or dieting does not affect the measure. The series includes 10 questions about food conditions of the household as a whole and of adults in the household and, if there are children present in the household, an additional 8 questions about their food conditions. The food security questions are listed in appendix A.

The food security status of each household is determined by the number of food-insecure conditions they report. Households are classified as *food secure* if they report no food-insecure conditions or if they report only one or two food-insecure conditions. They are classified as *food insecure* if they report three or more food-insecure conditions.

Food-insecure households are further classified as having either *low food security* or *very low food security*. Households classified as having *low food security* have reported multiple indications of food access problems and reductions in the quality or variety of their diets, but typically have reported few, if any, indications of reduced food intake. Households classified as having *very low food security* have reported multiple indications of reduced food intake and disrupted eating patterns due to inadequate resources for food.

WHAT ARE THE FOOD CONDITIONS IN HOUSEHOLDS WITH LOW AND VERY LOW FOOD SECURITY?

The responses of households in the December 2006 food security survey clearly reflect the difference between low and very low food security (figure 2). Households with *low food security* (about two-thirds of food-insecure households) reported mainly reductions in diet quality and variety (they could not afford to eat balanced meals) and difficulties and worries about food access. They typically report few if any indications of reductions in quantity of food intake.

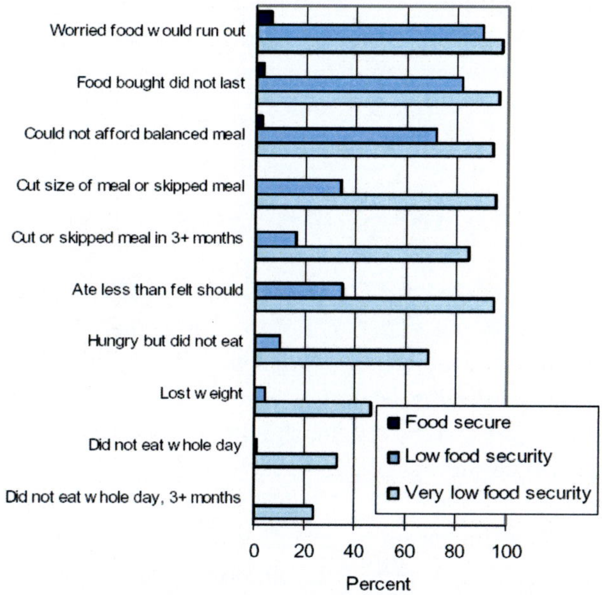

Source: Calculated by USDA, Economic Research Service using data from the December 2006 Current Population Survey Food Security Supplement.

Figure 2. Households reporting each indicator of food insecurity, by food security status, 2006.

The defining characteristic of *very low food security* is that, at times during the year, the food intake of household members is reduced and their normal eating patterns are disrupted because the household lacks money and other resources for food. Households classified as having very low food security in the 2006 survey reported the following specific conditions:

- 98 percent reported having worried that their food would run out before they got money to buy more.
- 96 percent reported that the food they bought just did not last and they did not have money to get more.
- 94 percent reported that they could not afford to eat balanced meals.
- 95 percent reported that an adult had cut the size of meals or skipped meals because there was not enough money for food.
- 85 percent reported that this had occurred in three or more months.
- In 95 percent, respondents reported that they had eaten less than they felt they should because there was not enough money for food.
- In 69 percent, respondents reported that they had been hungry but did not eat because they could not afford enough food.
- In 46 percent, respondents reported having lost weight because they did not have enough money for food.
- 33 percent reported that an adult did not eat for a whole day because there was not enough money for food.
- 24 percent reported that this had occurred in 3 or more months.

When interpreting food security statistics, it is important to keep in mind that households are classified as having low or very low food security if they experienced the condition at any time during the previous 12 months. The prevalence of these conditions on any given day is far below the corresponding annual prevalence.

How Does Food Insecurity Relate to Hunger?

Several years ago, USDA asked the Committee on National Statistics (CNSTAT) of the National Academies to convene an expert panel to ensure that the measurement methods used to assess households' access—or lack of access—to adequate food were conceptually and operationally sound. One of the central issues the CNSTAT panel addressed was the concept and definition of hunger and the relationship between hunger and food insecurity.

The CNSTAT panel recommended that USDA make a clear and explicit distinction between food insecurity and hunger. Food insecurity is a household-level economic and social condition of limited or uncertain access to adequate food. Hunger is an individual physiological condition that is a potential, although not inevitable, outcome of food insecurity. By measuring and monitoring food insecurity, USDA provides important information about the social and economic context in which hunger may occur, and contributes to the effective operation of the domestic nutrition assistance programs that provide millions of children and low-income people access to food, a healthful diet, and nutrition education.

HOUSEHOLD FOOD SECURITY IN THE UNITED STATES, 2006—A FEW MORE STATISTICS

Children in most food-insecure households—even in households with very low food security among adults—were protected from substantial reductions in food intake. However in about 221,000 households (0.6 percent of households with children) one or more children were also subject to reduced food intake and disrupted eating patterns at some time during the year (figure 3). In some households with very low food security among children, only older children may have been subjected to the more severe effects of food insecurity while younger children were protected from those effects.

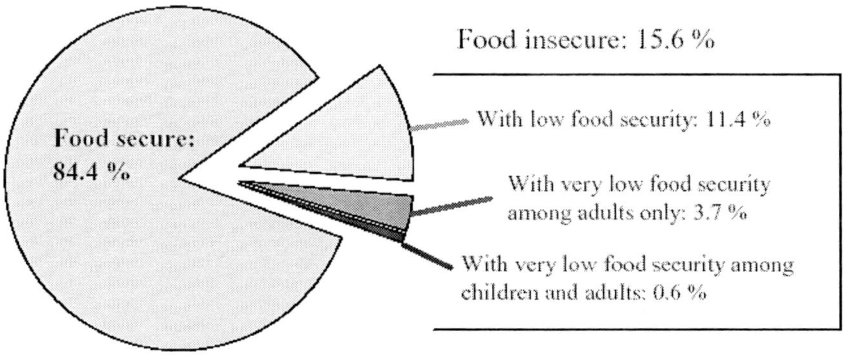

Source: Calculated by USDA, Economic Research Service using data from the December 2006 Current Population Survey Food Security Supplement.

Figure 3. Food security inU.S. households with children, 2006 (39.4 million households).

The prevalence of food insecurity varies considerably among different types of households. In 2006, rates of food insecurity were well below the national average for households with two or more adults and no children (6.5 percent) and for households with one or more members over the age of 65 (6.0 percent). Rates of food insecurity were substantially higher than the national average for households with incomes below the poverty line (36.3 percent), households with children headed by single women (30.4 percent) or single men (17.0 percent), and for Black and Hispanic households (21.8 percent and 19.5 percent, respectively).

Over the last decade, the prevalence of food insecurity has moved approximately in parallel with the national poverty rate, declining in the late 1 990s, increasing following the recession of 2001, and declining after 2004 (figure 4). The prevalence of very low food security has remained essentially unchanged since 2004.

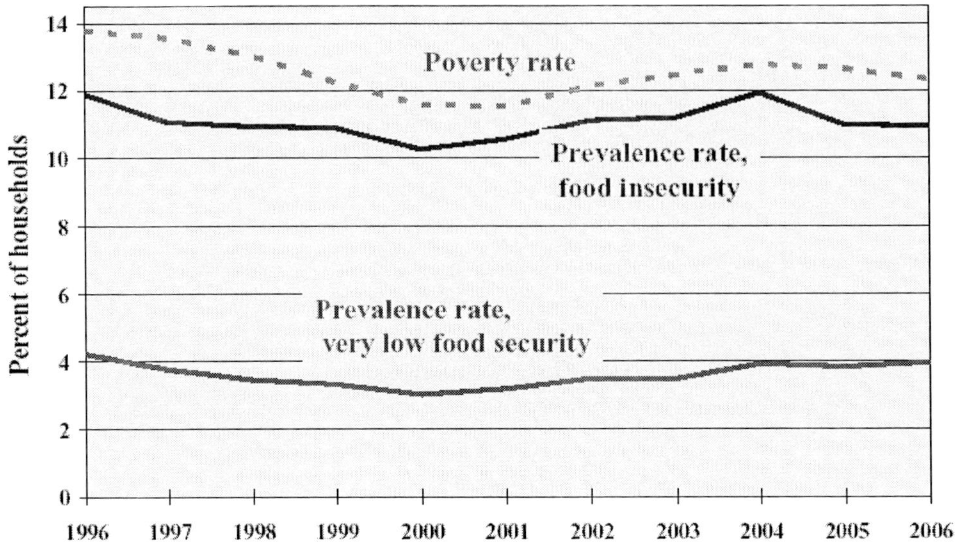

Note: Two-year rolling averages are presented for 1996-2001 to smooth seasonal fluctuations.
Source: Calculated by USDA, Economic Research Service using data from the December 2006 Current Population Survey Food Security Supplement.

Figure 4. Trends in food insecurity and poverty.

Mr. Chairman, this concludes my statement. I will be glad to answer questions the Committee may have.

APPENDIX A. QUESTIONS USED TO ASSESS THE FOOD SECURITY OF HOUSEHOLDS IN NATIONAL SURVEYS

1. "We worried whether our food would run out before we got money to buy more." Was that often, sometimes, or never true for you in the last 12 months?
2. "The food that we bought just didn't last and we didn't have money to get more." Was that often, sometimes, or never true for you in the last 12 months?
3. "We couldn't afford to eat balanced meals." Was that often, sometimes, or never true for you in the last 12 months?
4. In the last 12 months, did you or other adults in the household ever cut the size of your meals or skip meals because there wasn't enough money for food? (Yes/No)
5. (If yes to Question 4) How often did this happen—almost every month, some months but not every month, or in only 1 or 2 months?
6. In the last 12 months, did you ever eat less than you felt you should because there wasn't enough money for food? (Yes/No)
7. In the last 12 months, were you ever hungry, but didn't eat, because there wasn't enough money for food? (Yes/No)
8. In the last 12 months, did you lose weight because there wasn't enough money for food? (Yes/No)

9. In the last 12 months did you or other adults in your household ever not eat for a whole day because there wasn't enough money for food? (Yes/No)
10. (If yes to Question 9) How often did this happen—almost every month, some months but not every month, or in only 1 or 2 months?

(Questions 11-18 are asked only if the household included children age 0-18)

11. "We relied on only a few kinds of low-cost food to feed our children because we were running out of money to buy food." Was that often, sometimes, or never true for you in the last 12 months?
12. "We couldn't feed our children a balanced meal, because we couldn't afford that." Was that often, sometimes, or never true for you in the last 12 months?
13. "The children were not eating enough because we just couldn't afford enough food." Was that often, sometimes, or never true for you in the last 12 months?
14. In the last 12 months, did you ever cut the size of any of the children's meals because there wasn't enough money for food? (Yes/No)
15. In the last 12 months, were the children ever hungry but you just couldn't afford more food? (Yes/No)
16. In the last 12 months, did any of the children ever skip a meal because there wasn't enough money for food? (Yes/No)
17. (If yes to Question 16) How often did this happen—almost every month, some months but not every month, or in only 1 or 2 months?
18. In the last 12 months did any of the children ever not eat for a whole day because there wasn't enough money for food? (Yes/No)

Household food security status is determined by the number of food-insecure conditions reported. (Food-insecure conditions are indicated by responses of "often" or "sometimes" to questions 1-3 and 11-13, "almost every month" or "some months but not every month" to questions 5, 10, and 17, and "yes" to the other questions.)

Households are classified as *food secure* if they report no food-insecure conditions or if they report only one or two food-insecure conditions. They are classified as *food insecure* if they report three or more food-insecure conditions.

Food insecure households are further classified as having low or very low food security by the following criteria:

- For households with no child present, 3-5 food-insecure conditions indicates low food security and 6-10 indicates very low food security.
- For households with one or more children, 3-7 food-insecure conditions indicates low food security and 8-18 indicates very low food security. Five or more food-insecure conditions *among the children* (that is, in response to questions 11-18) indicates very low food security among chilren.

In: Hunger in America: Issues and Assistance
Editor: Gaston T. LaBue, pp. 133-138
ISBN: 978-1-60692-803-5

Chapter 7

Testimony before the Committee on Agriculture, Subcommittee on Department Operations, Oversight, Nutrition, and Forestry, United States House of Representatives, Hearing: The Short and Long Term Effects of Hunger in America, Wednesday, July 23, 2008

Diana Cutts*

Chairman Baca and distinguished members of the Committee, my name is Dr. Diana Cutts. I am honored to be given the opportunity to share with you my experience as a pediatrician and researcher at Hennepin County Medical Center (HCMC) in Minneapolis, Minnesota.

At HCMC my colleagues and I provide care for a diverse, urban population of children, including a significant immigrant population. I work in both out-patient and in-patient settings in a large general teaching hospital, usually supervising a team of bright young medical students, interns, and residents. I have special interest in pediatric nutritional problems and direct an interdisciplinary team of professionals devoted to the care of children who are not growing well. For the past fifteen years, I've also been involved in research on childhood hunger and I am a founder and principal investigator of the Children's Sentinel Nutrition Assessment Program (C-SNAP), a national, multi-site pediatric research program which focuses on the impact of public policies on babies and toddlers under the age of three years.

As I thought about how I could best add to the discussion today, I recognized the tremendous expertise and knowledge of those with whom I sit. And I concluded – with some relief - that I could rely on them to present specific policy information, while I could speak about a large part of what I do – take care of patients and teach trainees. So - I am going to

---

* www.c-snap. org

ask you all to join me on rounds as my team this morning, as I see children. Please place your stethoscopes around your necks, but don't bother with white coats – they only scare the kids.

Our first patient is Julia, a 13 month old who is seen following her recent three-day hospitalization for dehydration due to a stomach virus. You tell me her blood chemistries were markedly abnormal at admission, but normalized with IV fluids. Looking at the vital signs that the nurse has obtained, we see that she is regaining her weight though still underweight. In the exam room she begins to scream the minute she sees us, clutching her mother in fear. We examine her over her protests. Mom is told to bring her back for her well child visit in a few months. Her howls cease only as she is carried out of the clinic. Suddenly, the clinic is a lot quieter.

Second on our schedule is Terrance, a 4 year old here to complete forms for enrollment in Headstart. He's a busy pre-schooler, but does not pass the developmental screening today. His mother, 5 months pregnant, is also concerned and accepts our referral to the public schools for more extensive developmental evaluation. Together in the room, we talk with mom and I become concerned about mom's slightly withdrawn and flat affect. She admits yes, she's tired, but she's also a bit depressed. We talk about maternal depression and refer mom to mental health resources. As we come out of the room, we worry about whether mom has the energy to take care of Terrance, the baby, and herself. The smartest among you anticipate that I will want to know if you made sure that the family is enrolled in the WIC program.

As they leave for the lab to get Terrance's CBC and lead level, one of the CSNAP interviewers approaches me. "Dr. Cutts," she says, "I hope it was okay that I gave that family two bags of groceries." I explain to you that it is our practice to offer a bag of groceries to families who are surveyed for our CSNAP program, which has monitored the rate of household and child food security and other hardships in the clinic for the last 10 years. It turns out you have a background in political science and you ask me more about our findings. So I explain that although Minnesota is known as one of the top-ranking states for most health parameters, the home to a large number of international food corporations and a state with an overall state food insecurity rate of 8.2%, our hospital's rates of household food insecurity for families with children under three are the highest of any of the five CSNAP sites – 35% compared to an average of 15% for the Boston, Baltimore, Little Rock, and Philadelphia sites.

The CSNAP interviewer taps me again. "Dr. Cutts, I'm worried about that mom. She told me that she hasn't had much food for the last week because she was kicked out of her apartment building because the landlord couldn't pay the mortgage, and now she is living with some friends, and her WIC vouchers were lost when they moved, and..." Our morning is unraveling pretty fast – we contact the clinic social worker and try to get a message to mom in the lab to return to clinic so she can meet with him.

I turn to you to teach – Let's talk about the implications of food insecurity for her pregnancy and that not-yet-born child. Prenatal nutrition is essential to a healthy pregnancy, but poor maternal nutrition is associated with greater risk of prematurity, complications of delivery, and low birth weight which increase the likelihood of infant mortality, infant and child health problems, long-term developmental delays, and even chronic disease, such as heart disease and diabetes in adulthood.[1] In addition, maternal depression is more than two and a half times as likely in food insecure households.[2]

Depression impacts parenting in negative ways. We've offered mental health and visiting nurse services, we've ensured that Terrance and she stay enrolled in WIC, which will help protect his health and growth and her well-being[3] – is there more we should do?

What about Terrance's developmental delay? you ask, interrupting my litany.

I am impressed with your insightful question and will try to remember to give you high marks on your rotation evaluation– I tell you that C SNAP research has shown that very young children who live in food insecure households, even those meeting the level of only mild food insecurity, are two-thirds more likely to be at risk for cognitive, motor or socio-emotional problems on screening tests when compared to those living in food secure households.[4] Kindergarteners who are food insecure are more likely to have emotional and behavioral problems, too.[5] In older school-age children, we know that food can make a difference in school performance. Some of the strongest words of support for school breakfast programs have come from the school staff who provide time- out supervision for children who are disrupting a classroom. They tell us that a dramatic decrease in these behaviors follows institution of breakfast programs, in addition to improved school attendance and improved standardized test scores.[6]

At any rate, it's probably not a coincidence that this particular child, whose mother described serious food insecurity, failed our screening. Developmental services to toddlers and pre-schoolers are the beginning of a societal cost of food insecurity that may be carried on into school years and throughout a lifetime of economic and social difficulties and diminished potential[7]

Even I'm getting tired of my long-winded responses to your questions now and the nurse is getting worried about us being behind schedule. I wisely decide to split you all up to send you each into the rooms of the remaining waiting patients.

And I sit down for a breather.

I think of the earlier patient we saw:

The little screamer, Julia, her family seemed okay, but I know from my own local data that children of color, like Julia, are at highest risk for food insecurity. Poor nutrition is an important contributor to the health disparities that are seen in children of color[8] as well as poor children compared to more privileged children. Children from food insecure households are 30% more likely to be hospitalized because of their diminished reserve and vulnerability in the face of typical childhood illnesses.[9] An average pediatric hospitalization for a child under three costs approximately $1 1,300[10], so, at least in part, these medical costs are actually another societal economic cost of food insecurity. These kids can't just bounce back because their immune systems are depressed from inadequate nutrition and they often begin a cycle of weight loss and recurrent infections that then perpetuate each other. I'll have to keep a close eye on Julia's growth at the next visit. Could Julia's hospitalization have been avoided if she was living in a more food secure environment? Oh, and was she well-insured? Would hospital bills further erode the family's ability to put nutritious food on the table?

I take a look at the schedule which tells me which patients you are each seeing.

One of you is doing a follow-up for anemia in six month old twins. Young children in food insecure households are two and a half times more likely to have iron-deficiency anemia as children in food secure households.[11] And iron deficiency anemia influences young children's brain development in detrimental ways, affecting attention, memory and language and social ability as well as depressing their immune systems. Gotta check in with mom about food security and watch their development carefully as I see them at future visits.

Someone else is interviewing Stephanie, a 14 year old whom I've known since she was 3 years old. She's struggled with childhood obesity since infancy, really, and her last recorded weight was 278 pounds. She began refusing to be weighed 2 years ago, so there's no weight recorded today by the nurse. She's had surgery to remove her tonsils and adenoids because of obstructive sleep apnea, a well-recognized complication of obesity. And she complains of chronic back pain, among other medical complaints. More threatening to her current well-being, her behavior's become out of control – she's sampling every imaginable risky behavior and not attending her alternative school. She's even admitted to suicidal thoughts.[12] I recall how CSNAP data obtained from this family years ago revealed the most severe food insecurity the interviewer had ever encountered – and our subsequent discussion about the apparent paradox of obesity co-existing with food insecurity due in great part to tight food budgets forcing parents to choose low-cost foods, which are mostly high in calories and very poor in nutrition.[13] Many years later, we still have a long way to go to help people understand this, and to impart the message that a piece of the response to the obesity epidemic must be to address food insecurity.

We end our morning with Brandon, a five year old with a cough, and his grandmother. He tells me a knock-knock joke. You tell me he has a history of asthma and, in fact, was hospitalized three weeks ago for an asthma attack and pneumonia. He was in the hospital for four days, but his grandmother reports he was okay until two days ago, when his cough re-appeared. I'm surprised when she tells me that he's not on any medicines. She explains to me that the family was not able to afford to fill the prescriptions that were given to them at hospital discharge, stating the charge to them was well over $100, and that they needed the money for food, the gas bill, and rent. We work out a plan to provide the needed medications, and hopefully prevent another hospitalization, while still preserving food security, energy access, and housing.

It's time to dismiss you all for your noon conference while I face the chart documentation and a stack of phone messages that I need to get to.

Do all of my patients' ills stem from food insecurity? Of course not. But, my reality is that for more than a third of them, food insecurity is a constant companion to their health, directly and indirectly influencing it in both immediate and distant ways. None of these children, who each came to clinic for a different reason, had a placard around their neck or a physical sign identifying them as food insecure. They are simply the typical pediatric patients seen daily all over this country in medical clinics serving low-income populations. 29 million children in this country are considered low-income, nearly 40% of our citizens less than 18 years old.[14]

These are the faces of child hunger in the United States, very different from the visibly starved Appalachian babies I saw in Life magazine when I was growing up, but no less real, no less impactful. Food insecurity in childhood changes the trajectory of young lives in a real and significant way. The quality of our communities is impacted, and there are high, and rising, economic costs which we all bear.

I feel privileged to play a role in creating a healthy and bright future for the children I see at HCMC. But my reach as their doctor is typically one child, one family at a time. Your reach spans the country and I urge you to think of our time together in clinic and boldly work to create programs and policies that promote healthy and bright futures for all children. For example, I know that Congress is considering another economic stimulus package; I encourage you to make a temporarily increased food stamp benefit part of the package, as it would do so much to directly help the children I've just told you about.

Nutrition assistance programs, such as the Food Stamp Program and WIC, are the medicines needed to treat food insecurity and these accompanying illnesses, but the programs need to be dosed at levels that cure rather than just diminish the problem. The programs are also critical and economically sound investments on the health end of the equation, as they provide the physiological building blocks necessary for proper growth, health, development, and learning. Better still would be a society in which an adequate, nutritious diet is achievable for every child without targeted intervention programs. Until that day comes, preventive efforts are the best way to avoid the tangible and long-lasting costs of food insecurity in childhood. Other programs that assist low-income families with basic needs that compete with the food budget, such as housing, energy, and childcare assistance, are equally vital, particularly in our current economic climate of rising food and energy prices.

No child deserves to be burdened with the consequences of this fully preventable condition for the duration of his/her life, and no responsible, far-sighted society should permit the widespread incidence of a condition like food insecurity that is guaranteed to produce a less healthy, capable, and productive population.

Class dismissed. Thank you.

References

[1] Cook JT and Frank DA. Food Security, Poverty, and Human Development in the United States. *Ann. N.Y. Acad. Sci.* 2008; xxxx: 1–16.

[2] Casey P, Goolsby S, Berkowitz C et. al,Maternal Depression, Changing Public Assistance, Food Security, and Child Health Status. *Pediatrics*. 2004; 113(2):298-304.

[3] Black M, Cutts D, Frank DA et al, Special Supplemental Nutrition Program for Women, Infants, and Children (WIC) Participation and Infants' Growth and Health: A Multisite Surveillance Study. *Pediatrics.* 2004: 114(1):169-176.

[4] Rose-Jacobs R, Black M, Casey P, et. al. Household food insecurity: Associations with at-risk infant and toddler development. *Pediatrics* 2008; 121:65-72.

[5] Stormer A and Harrison GG. Does household food insecurity affect cognitive and social development of kindergarteners? *California Center for Population Research*, University of California—Los Angeles, November 2003.

[6] Minnesota Department of Children, Families & Learning, Fast Break to Learning – 1999-2000 Executive Summary and Meals for Learning 2000 Report.

[7] Murphy C, Ettinger de Cuba S, Cook, J et al. Economic Costs of Food Insecurity for Young Children: A Report from the Children's Sentinel Nutrition Assessment Program (C-SNAP) and the Food Research and Action Center (FRAC). Commissioned by the *Partnership for America's Economic Success and Pew Charitable Trusts*. Forthcoming October 2008.

[8] The Impact of Food Insecurity on the Development of Young Low-Income Black and Latino Children; and Protecting the Health and Nutrition of Young Children of

Color: The Impact of Nutrition Assistance and Income Support Programs. Research Findings from the Children's Sentinel Nutrition Assessment Program (C-SNAP); Prepared for the Joint Center for Political and Economic Studies Health Policy Institute, May 2006.

[9] Cook JT, Frank DA, Berkowitz C, et al. Food Insecurity is Associated with Adverse Health Outcomes Among Human Infants and Toddlers. *Journal of Nutrition.* 2004; 134:1432-1438.

[10] Children's Sentinel Nutrition Assessment Program unpublished data (excluding costs associated with birth), 2007.

[11] Skalicky A, Meyers A, Adams W, et al. Child Food Insecurity and Iron Deficiency Anemia in Low- Income Infants and Toddlers in the United States. *Maternal and Child Health Journal*. 2006;10(2):177- 185.

[12] Falkner, N.H. et. al. Social, educational, and psychological correlates of weight status in adolescents. *Obesity Research.* 2001; 9(1):32-42.

[13] Drewnowski, A. and S.E. Specter. Poverty and obesity: The role of energy density and energy costs. *Am. J. Clin. Nutr*. 2004;79(1):6-16.

[14] National Center for Children in Poverty. Poverty 101. http://www.nccp.org/faq.html Accessed July 20, 2008.

In: Hunger in America: Issues and Assistance
Editor: Gaston T. LaBue, pp. 139-142
ISBN: 978-1-60692-803-5

Chapter 8

TESTIMONY BEFORE THE U.S. HOUSE OF REPRESENTATIVES COMMITTEE ON AGRICULTURE, SUBCOMMITTEE ON DEPARTMENT OPERATIONS, OVERSIGHT, NUTRITION AND FORESTRY

J. Larry Brown

July 23, 2008

Mr. Chairman,
Members of the Committee:

I thank you for your invitation to appear today as you consider the health and economic costs of hunger in America. Although I have appeared before this and other Committees on many occasions over the years, I must begin with the bottom line: The United States is quite unique among industrial democracies because we let so many of our people go hungry, and we seem to be doing precious little to close this gap. Year after year the Department reports that about 35 million Americans live in households that do not have enough to eat. What was once termed a "hunger epidemic" in our nation has now become a continuing fact of life. We are letting this problem remain pretty much the same from year to year. Clearly we can do better, and I applaud you for holding this hearing to exercise the leadership to make a difference.

Before I turn to the results of our study of the cost burden of hunger, I will begin by reviewing what science knows about the health and cognitive effects of hunger—what it does to the minds and bodies of both children and adults. Some of this information may be new to you, even to the two Members who also are physicians by training.

Two or three decades ago I used to teach my public health and medical students that while hunger impacts one's health status, it seldom had an effect on the brain. We now know that this is not true. Science now knows that there is no "safe" level of hunger: when a child is forced to go without enough to eat her body suffers and her brain function is impaired. The same is true for adults, particularly the vulnerable elderly. This is because the body and the brain require sufficient food energy to function adequately. When it is not there, even temporarily, the body and mind cannot function properly. Just as your car cannot run without the proper fuel, so too is the mind impaired when it goes without its own fuel.

A child sitting in the classroom without a breakfast does not have the cognitive capacity to take part in the educational process. Her body is in the classroom but her mind is not fueled to learn. This is because when the body does not have enough nourishment, even on a short-term basis, it goes into triage. Just like triage on the battlefield, the body must decide how to allocate its insufficient resources. Its first priority is to use whatever energy there is to maintain critical organ function. Its next priority, if there is enough nutrient energy, is to maintain health. Its final priority is for brain function. As my colleague Carl Sagan bluntly put it when we discussed these new research findings, "better dumb than dead." That child in the class may be present in body but she came through the schoolhouse door too impaired to learn—not because she is dumb but because she suffers cognitive impairment due to lack of nutrition. In short, science now knows that hunger, not just in its absolute state but even in the form of chronically "mild" under-nutrition, produces startling effects in both the mind and body. While true for both adults and children, most of the research has focused on the young because we can more easily track their growth and educational patterns. Children without enough to eat:

- Get sick more frequently, particularly in terms of preventable outcomes such headaches, stomachaches and colds,
- They have more difficulty overcoming illnesses once they occur,
- They miss school more often due to these illnesses,
- They have more behavioral disorders, such as aggressiveness and classroom disruption, as well as sullen and withdrawn behavior, and
- They do less well in terms of their grades and do more poorly on standardized test scores than do similar children who get enough to eat.

It is in the context of these poorer health, behavioral and mental outcomes that the Sodexo Foundation commissioned me, along with three other scholars, to assess their cost to the nation. In other words, how much more money do we pay in terms of illness, poor educational outcomes and lost productivity than we would if no one went hungry in America. I am joined today by one of my colleagues in this research, Dr. Don Shepard, an economist from Brandeis University, who has done similar cost burden analyses, recently one commissioned by the United Nations regarding the cost of dengue fever. Sodexo, known for its corporate interest not only charitable responses to hunger but to informed policy responses to help end hunger altogether, funded our interdisciplinary team from three major universities. Parenthetically, I should mention that none of us receives a salary from Sodexo, and the Foundation played no role whatsoever in our research or its outcomes.

When people go hungry it costs the nation in a variety of ways, some of which are not easily measurable. We dismissed cost areas for which calculations were too difficult, and focused instead on four key cost arenas that are more easily measurable, that is, where the scientific literature is sufficient to develop cost burdens that are both reasonable and conservative. The first of these is charity. It is said that "there is no free lunch."

Somebody, somewhere, pays. Charity operates the same way, and hunger charities exist throughout the country, in each of your districts and in virtually every community in the nation. More than 300 food banks exist, covering every state and averaging six to a state (although they are not that equally distributed). These food banks provide nutritional and other commodities to more than 50,000 soup kitchens and food pantries. These food banks and local charities have to rent or purchase offices, warehouses, freezers, trucks and related materials. They have to have full-time, paid staff, and their work is supplemented by literally thousands upon thousands of volunteers who often spend from several hours to a day or two a week helping to feed the hungry. Each of these activities, even among volunteers, has a cost. We figured out what it is. This enormous charitable enterprise comes to more than $14.5 billion each year.

We next turn to the excess cost of illness, that is, illness that is associated with hunger over and above the typical levels that occur in the population(s). We did this for both mental health services and for medical and other forms of health care. You might be interested in how we did this. As indicated earlier, we know that food-deprived groups have higher rates of ill health: iron deficiency occurs at a rate that is 1.66 times more likely; activity-limiting health impairments are nearly three times as high; headaches nearly twice as high; and nutrient deficiencies from three to four times normal levels. In terms of mental health outcomes, particularly in children, depression is 3.5 times higher than among non-hungry children; the need for special education twice as high; and general psychosocial dysfunction is seven times as high. As you're probably beginning to see, it costs far less to feed children than it is to let them go hungry and par a higher price after-the-fact. I will go no further now in terms of how we attributed actual costs of these adverse outcomes, but Dr. Shepard and I can take questions, or you can refer to the detailed methodology in our research report. What is worth noting now is that the health-related costs of hunger come to nearly $67 billion annually. And please bear in mind that the actual costs certainly are higher, quite a bit higher, because of our conservative methodology. This is because for some outcomes, say Attention Deficit Hyperactivity Disorder (ADHD), the research literature is insufficient to develop likelihood ratios for excess outcomes. For yet other outcomes, we had adequate data to compute direct costs but not for indirect ones. It is the responsibility of researchers to be careful— conservative— and it is for this reason that we know our estimate of $67 billion a year does not capture the full cost in this arena.

The final cost arena is the limited education and lowered workforce productivity that is associated with having too little nourishment. According to a number of studies in this field, children from food insecure homes are more likely than their non-hungry peers to do less well on tests of mental ability and overall school performance. They miss school 50% more; they get suspended about twice as often; and they have to repeat more grades. They also are less likely to complete high school. As a result, children so affected face greater likelihood of unemployment or limited employment; poor judgment and lowered job performance; and, as a result, lowered workforce productivity. The cost of this productivity loss comes to $9.2 billion annually.

When we add the costs of each of these arenas (more than $14 billion for charity; nearly $67 billion for illness; and almost $10 billion in lowered education and productivity) we pay a rather staggering bill for hunger-- more than $90 billion each year. This is enough to get our attention, although I stress again that the actual cost is clearly higher than this, due to our utilization of conservative research techniques and lack of sufficient data for some outcomes known to be associated with hunger.

While this bill, sort of an additional tax on the American public, is not evenly distributed across the population, it means that a typical household in our country pays $500 a year. While this bill often is not direct, it shows up in terms of higher taxes to cover the costs of outcomes that the victims of hunger suffer. It also is paid in terms of charitable contributions and related tax deductions, as well as lowered workforce productivity and competitiveness in the international market system.

By contrast to this $90 billion annual cost, it recently was estimated that we could virtually end hunger in America if we increased spending for existing nutrition programs (food stamps, school meals, summer feeding and elderly feeding) by about $12 billion a year over current spending. (The very recent jump in food and fuel costs may now make this calculation somewhat higher).

Former nutrition advisor to President Nixon, Dr. Jean Mayer, once noted that "of all the dumb ways to save money, not feeding children is the dumbest." While I prefer to speak a slightly different language than his remarkable clarity, our economics are clear: our nation pays far more to let hunger exist than it would cost us to eliminate it.

Thank you.

Copies of the research analysis, The Economic Cost of Domestic Hunger: Estimated Annual Burden to the United States, *is available to download by going to www.sodexofoundation.com. For further information from the researchers, email: lbrown@hsph.harvard.edu; shepard@brandeis.edu; martin@brandeis.edu; and orwat@loyola.edu. This research initiative was sponsored by Sodexo Foundation, which has been working to eliminate the root causes of hunger since 1996. Its work also includes a broad menu of child feeding programs (summer and school year), and disaster response initiatives such as Hurricane Katrina and the Gulf Coast.*

INDEX

A

D

E

F

G

H

O

P

Q

R

S

T

U

V

W

Y